OXFORD MEDICAL PUBLICATIONS

Heart Failure

Oxford Specialist Handbooks published and forthcoming

General Oxford Specialist Handbooks
A Resuscitation Room Guide
Addiction Medicine
Perioperative Medicine,
Second Edition
Post-Operative Complications,
Second edition

Oxford Specialist Handbooks in Anaesthesia
Cardiac Anaesthesia
General Thoracic Anaesthesia
Neuroanaesthesia
Obstetric Anaesthesia
Paediatric Anaesthesia
Regional Anaesthesia, Stimulation and Ultrasound Techniques

Oxford Specialist Handbooks in Cardiology
Adult Congenital Heart Disease
Cardiac Catheterization and Coronary Intervention
Echocardiography
Fetal Cardiology
Heart Failure
Hypertension
Nuclear Cardiology
Pacemakers and ICDs

Oxford Specialist Handbooks in Critical Care
Advanced Respiratory Critical Care

Oxford Specialist Handbooks in End of Life Care
Cardiology
Dementia
Nephrology
Respiratory Disease
The Intensive Care Unit

Oxford Specialist Handbooks in Neurology
Epilepsy
Parkinson's Disease and Other Movement Disorders
Stroke Medicine

Oxford Specialist Handbooks in Paediatrics
Paediatric Endocrinology and Diabetes
Paediatric Dermatology
Paediatric Gastroenterology, Hepatology, and Nutrition
Paediatric Haematology and Oncology
Paediatric Nephrology
Paediatric Neurology
Paediatric Radiology
Paediatric Respiratory Medicine

Oxford Specialist Handbooks in Psychiatry
Child and Adolescent Psychiatry
Old Age Psychiatry

Oxford Specialist Handbooks in Radiology
Interventional Radiology
Musculoskeletal Imaging

Oxford Specialist Handbooks in Surgery
Cardiothoracic Surgery
Hand Surgery
Hepato-pancreatobiliary Surgery
Oral Maxillo Facial Surgery
Neurosurgery
Operative Surgery, Second Edition
Otolaryngology and Head and Neck Surgery
Plastic and Reconstructive Surgery
Surgical Oncology
Urological Surgery
Vascular Surgery

Heart Failure
From advanced disease to bereavement

Miriam Johnson

Reader in Palliative Medicine
Hull York Medical School (HYMS)
Honorary Consultant in Palliative Medicine to
St Catherine's Hospice

Karen Hogg

Consultant Cardiologist
Glasgow Royal Infirmary and
Golden Jubilee National Hospital

James Beattie

Consultant Cardiologist
Heart of England NHS Foundation Trust Birmingham and
National Clinical Lead NHS Improvement—Heart

Series Editor
Max Watson

Consultant
Northern Ireland Hospice, Belfast
Honorary Consultant
Princess Alice Hospice, Esher
Visiting Professor
University of Ulster, Belfast

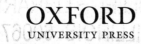

OXFORD
UNIVERSITY PRESS

OXFORD
UNIVERSITY PRESS

Great Clarendon Street, Oxford OX2 6DP
United Kingdom

Oxford University Press is a department of the University of Oxford.
It furthers the University's objective of excellence in research, scholarship,
and education by publishing worldwide. Oxford is a registered trade mark of
Oxford University Press in the UK and in certain other countries

British Library Cataloguing in Publication Data
Data available

Library of Congress Cataloging in Publication Data
Library of Congress Control Number: 2011944044

ISBN 978-0-19-929930-0

Printed in Great Britain
on acid-free paper by
Ashford Colour Press Ltd, Gosport, Hampshire

Oxford University Press makes no representation, express or implied, that the
drug dosages in this book are correct. Readers must therefore always check
the product information and clinical procedures with the most up-to-date
published product information and data sheets provided by the manufacturers
and the most recent codes of conduct and safety regulations. The authors and
the publishers do not accept responsibility or legal liability for any errors in the
text or for the misuse or misapplication of material in this work. Except where
otherwise stated, drug dosages and recommendations are for the non-pregnant
adult who is not breast-feeding

Links to third party websites are provided by Oxford in good faith and
for information only. Oxford disclaims any responsibility for the materials
contained in any third party website referenced in this work.

Contents

Detailed contents

Contributors

Dr Miriam Johnson
Reader in Palliative Medicine
Hull York Medical School (HYMS)
Honorary Consultant in Palliative
Medicine to St Catherine's
Hospice

Dr Karen Hogg
Consultant Cardiologist
Glasgow Royal Infirmary and
Golden Jubilee National Hospital

Dr James Beattie
Consultant Cardiologist
Heart of England NHS Foundation
Trust Birmingham and
National Clinical Lead NHS
Improvement—Heart

Series Editor
Dr Max Watson
Consultant
Northern Ireland Hospice, Belfast
Honorary Consultant
Princess Alice Hospice, Esher
Visiting Professor
University of Ulster, Belfast

Additional contributions by:

Dr Shona Jenkins
SpR Cardiology
Glasgow Royal Infirmary

Dr Suzanne Kite MA FRCP
Consultant in Palliative Medicine
The Leeds Teaching Hospitals
NHS Trust

Mrs Annie MacCallum
Professional Lead for Specialist
Nursing Services
NHS Gloucestershire Care
Services

Acknowledgement

The chapters on Diagnosing end-stage heart disease (Chapter 5), Management of pain (Chapter 9), and Spiritual and religious care (Chapter 14) include adapted text from *End of Life Care in Nephrology: From Advanced Disease to Bereavement* by Edwina Brown, E Joanna Chambers and Celia Eggeling, Oxford University Press, 2007. With permission of Oxford University Press.

Symbols and abbreviations

📖	cross-reference in this book
AAs	aldosterone antagonists
ACE	angiotensin-converting enzyme
ACP	advance care planning
ADL	activities of daily living
ADRT	advance decision to refuse treatment
A&E	Accident and Emergency [hospital department]
AF	atrial fibrillation
ARBs	angiotensin II receptor antagonists
AV	atrioventricular [node]
B3G	buprenorphine-3-glucuronide
bd	twice a day
BHF	British Heart Foundation
BiVAD	biventricular assist device
BMA	British Medical Association
BNP	brain natriuretic peptide
BP	blood pressure
CABG	coronary artery bypass graft
CNS	central nervous system
COPD	chronic obstructive pulmonary disease
CPR	cardiopulmonary resuscitation
CrCL	creatinine clearance
CRT	cardiac resynchronization therapy [device]
CRTD	cardiac resynchronization therapy [device] with defibrillator
CRTP	CRT [with] pacemaker
DCM	dilated cardiomyopathy
DIG	Digitalis Investigation Group
DNACPR	do not attempt cardiopulmonary resuscitation
DVT	deep vein thrombosis
ECG	electrocardiogram
ESAS	Edmonton Symptom Assessment Scale
FPA	financial power of attorney
GMC	General Medical Council [UK]
GP	general practitioner
GSF	Gold Standards Framework

H3G	hydromorphone-3-glucuronide
HF	heart failure
HFNS	heart failure nurse specialist
HFSS	Heart Failure Survival Score
H-ISDN	hydralazine and isosorbide dinitrate
HIV	human immunodeficiency virus
hr	hour(s)
HRUK	Heart Rhythm UK
ICD	implantable cardioverter defibrillator
IABP	intra-aortic balloon pump
IV	intravenous
KCCQ	Kansas City Cardiomyopathy Questionnaire
KPS	Karnofsky Performance Status/Score
LCP	Liverpool Care Pathway [for the Dying]
LMWH	low molecular weight heparin
LPA	lasting power of attorney
LV	left ventricle
LVAD	left ventricular assist device
LVEF	left ventricular ejection fraction
M3G	morphine-3-glucuronide
M6G	morphine-6-glucuronide
mcg	microgram
mg	milligram
MI	myocardial infarction
MR	mitral regurgitation
MV	mitral valve
NaSSA	noradrenergic and specific serotonergic antidepressant
NICE	National Institute for Health and Clinical Excellence
NMDA	*N-methyl-D-aspartate*
NNT	number needed to treat
nocte	at night
NorB	norbuprenorphine
NRS	numerical rating scale
NSAID	non-steroidal anti-inflammatory drug
NYHA	New York Heart Association
od	once a day
OOH	out of hours
PCI	percutaneous coronary intervention
POA	power of attorney
PPA	property power of attorney

PPS	post-phlebitic syndrome
prn	as needed
qds	four times a day
RAAS	renin–angiotensin–aldosterone system
SARI	serotonin antagonist and re-uptake inhibitor
SC	subcutaneous
SHFS	Seattle Heart Failure Score
SL	sublingual
SNRI	serotonin–norepinephrine re-uptake inhibitor
SSRI	selective serotonin re-uptake inhibitor
TD	transdermal
tds	three times a day
VAD	ventricular assist device
VF	ventricular fibrillation
VO2max	maximal oxygen consumption
VT	ventricular tachycardia
WHO	World Health Organization
WPA	health/welfare power of attorney

The challenge of patients with heart failure (HF): barriers to accessing supportive and palliative care

Introduction

HF is a major public health problem, which is escalating due to the aging population, improved survival rates from acute cardiac syndromes, and the impact of secondary prevention. Therapy for HF has increased survival and improved symptoms.

Potential therapeutic strategies for HF include:[1-3]

- Conventional drug therapy.
- Complex device therapy:
  - implantable cardioverter defibrillator (ICD)
  - cardiac resynchronization therapy (CRT).
- Ventricular assist devices.
- Cardiac transplantation.

However, symptom burden and mortality remain high, and for many quality of life is poor on a scale similar to or worse than for many common cancers. Despite this, patients with HF still lack routine access to palliative care services.[3-6] Patients in developed countries tend to be elderly (average age 76) with concomitant comorbidities and psychosocial problems associated with age and chronic disease.[3,7] Failure to address the supportive and palliative care needs of this patient group risks the following:

- Persistent symptom burden.
- Prolonged caregiver burden.
- Loss of opportunity to be involved in planning for end of life care.
- Risk of inappropriate and most often prolonged hospital admissions.
- Risk of inappropriate and unwanted hospital death.

These unmet needs are well known but barriers exist that until recently have deterred the provision of palliative care for people with HF. However, although challenging, providing this type of care and service has been deemed an international public health priority.[8,9]

Barriers to accessing supportive and palliative care

Barriers can be divided into three main groups: general, cardiological, and palliative care.

General barriers

- Poor understanding from patients, families, health care professionals, and the general public about the inevitable consequences of HF, including the likelihood of disease progression and death.
- Lack of appreciation of the need for palliative care and/or the potential advantages.
- Health care professionals and patients are often unclear what palliative care or hospices have to offer in terms of HF management.
- Negative connotations surrounding palliative care, hospices, and the associated terminology. Palliative care services and hospices are associated by many with malignancy or imminent death. As such, referral to palliative care services is made harder for the health professional and the patient to accept.
- Patients may be disheartened, having been told that there are no further treatment options, or socially isolated and/or depressed, leaving them less likely to consider other opportunities unless presented to them in an accessible way.

Consequently many patients may not consider, or be unable to cope with, referral to palliative care services unless this is discussed with skill and sensitivity; this situation may also be seen in patients with malignancy, where it appears to be less of a barrier. Rather than address the issues outlined above, many health care professionals merely make the assumption that HF patients would not wish referral to palliative care.

Cardiological barriers

Unpredictable disease trajectory

The clinical course of HF is one of slow decline interspersed with intermittent serious deteriorations from which the patient, at least initially, may recover from to be almost, but not quite, as well as they were before. The deteriorations may be difficult to predict, and it may also be difficult to predict which deterioration will lead to death (see Box 1.1). In contrast, the clinical course for many people with cancer can run a more predictable pattern.

This clinical course is called the 'disease trajectory' (◻ Chapter 3) and the unpredictable nature of the HF trajectory is cited as one of the main barriers to recognizing advanced disease and accessing supportive and palliative care services for such people.

With HF there may be no clear point at which the patient no longer responds to treatment and moves into the palliative phase. This is discussed more fully in ◻ Chapters 3 and 6.

Box 1.1 Factors contributing to the unpredictability of the HF illness trajectory

- Multiple and unpredictable hospital admissions due to clinical decompensation.
- Many patients recover from these episodes; sophisticated techniques are now available to help patients stabilize in the acute setting.
- Some HF strategies, such as CRT, may improve the patient's quality of life and symptoms thus temporarily reversing the disease trajectory for a period of time.
- Although the risk of sudden cardiac death has reduced with the use of ICDs and the systematic use of beta-blockers, this is still an issue for those who are not eligible for, or who do not wish to have, these interventions.
- There is no validated scoring mechanism that can adequately identify the individual potentially most in need of a palliative approach.
- Unlike patients with cancer, HF patients are not always managed by a specialist.
- Non-cardiologists looking after HF patients, including primary care practitioners, may not feel confident that all treatment options have been exhausted and adopt the 'wait and see approach'.
- Cardiologists may find it difficult to discern when available treatment options are no longer appropriate and that the focus should be on symptom management.

Thus faced with such an unpredictable illness trajectory the tendency for health professionals is to continue with traditional therapeutic strategies for HF in an attempt to stabilize the patient and not consider palliative care. Patients often feel that as they have survived one episode of decompensation they could survive again; so the revolving door cycle of hospital admissions and clinical decompensation episodes continues.

Lack of skills and knowledge
In addition, symptom control, end of life care for patients, and advanced communication skills are not part of the curriculum for cardiology trainees. There is, in general, also a lack of knowledge regarding primary care services that can support patients in their own homes if that is their preferred place of care.

Poor communication and co-ordination of services
Although the ethos of multidisciplinary team working is improving, this rarely crosses the primary/secondary care divide. The following may affect clarity regarding a patient's stage of disease:
- Pressure on hospital beds may mitigate against a wider assessment being made, and the patient is discharged home as soon as fluid balance is restored without plans for future care.
- Repeated hospital admissions may be under the care of various consultants and a connected overview may not occur.
- Communication from secondary care to primary care may not include an assessment of the current stage of illness in the context of the overall stage of illness and an indication of the most appropriate management.

- Although clinicians in primary care may be well placed to discuss these issues with the patient, they may not have the confidence to do so without clear support from their secondary care colleagues.
- Hospital outpatient clinics are rarely organized to accommodate complex patients with multidomain issues that require careful and sensitive discussion.

Palliative care barriers

The traditional view of chronic disease management and palliative care, whereby chronic disease management needs to end before palliative care management can start, is described more fully in ☐ Chapter 3. This understanding of care acts as a barrier to providing supportive and palliative care parallel to and integrated with traditional HF therapies; this more appropriate concept is driven by a problem approach to care rather than one based on prognosis, and is outlined in ☐ Chapters 6 and 7.

Further issues relating to palliative care services may act as a barrier for people with HF:

- Palliative care originated in the voluntary sector funded by cancer charities.
- Many current palliative care services are funded through cancer charities such as Macmillan Cancer Relief and Marie Curie Cancer Care.
- Many palliative care professionals have had most experience with malignant disease, and understandably have concerns regarding general medical knowledge, exacerbated by the advancing complexity of available evidence-based therapies.
- There is no history of joint working or training between the two specialties.
- There are concerns about saturating an already stretched service, with fears that the unpredictable illness trajectory makes service planning difficult and worries that valuable inpatient hospice beds may be blocked by patients with debilitating disease but who are not in imminent danger of death.
- Some hospices run by cancer charities may have restricted purpose and be unable to accept people with non-malignant disease.

'Prognostic paralysis'

The end result of these barriers is the all too common situation of 'prognostic paralysis'[10,11] where neither clinician nor patient recognizes the transition to advanced disease and the need for supportive and palliative care. Patients therefore miss out on:

- The opportunity to receive optimal symptom assessment and management supports (social, psychological, financial, and spiritual) for both them and their family or carer.
- Opportunities to discuss end of life decisions including resuscitation, defibrillator deactivation, preferred place of care, and planning for care at the end of life.

The almost inevitable consequence of this path is recurrent hospital admissions leading up to death in hospital.

This book aims to help the clinician to recognize and appropriately manage advanced, end-stage disease, and the patient who is now dying.

Case example: a situation to avoid. . .

Adrian is a 68-year-old married man with two adult children. He has had New York Heart Association (NYHA) class III–IV HF for 10 years. A cardiac resynchronization therapy with defibrillator (CRTD) device was inserted just over a year ago. He has been reasonably well until the last 6–8 months, but now:

- Worsening renal impairment (urea 32mmol/L, creatinine 436µmol/L).
- Intolerance of angiotensin-converting enzyme (ACE) inhibitors and spironolactone which had to be stopped.
- Five protracted admissions to hospital with HF and recurrent episodes of ventricular tachycardia (VT) appropriately treated with shock therapy from his CRTD device.
- Is house bound with increasing time spent in bed asleep.
- Is cachectic.

Despite this, he, his wife, and his two children did not realize he was seriously unwell. During his final admission with pulmonary oedema he developed VT requiring multiple shocks. He was managed with several attempts to place a central line and monitor arterial blood gases, intravenous (IV) furosemide, IV amiodarone, and 32 shocks from an external defibrillator during attempted cardiopulmonary resuscitation (CPR). He died in hospital without his family.

Case example: better way?

Jim, aged 78, had NYHA class III–IV HF with an ICD in place. Over 4–6 months his condition deteriorated with:

- Four prolonged hospital admissions precipitated by pulmonary oedema and appropriate shocks from his ICD for VT.
- An unsuccessful VT ablation.
- Tolerance of only sub-optimal doses of his HF therapy.

During his final admission, he had four appropriate shocks from his ICD for VT. However, he became progressively nauseated and anorectic, with resistant fluid overload and mild hypokalaemia. He was managed with IV diuretics initially, but switched to high-dose oral diuretics when the IV route became distressing. He was given laxatives for constipation, anti-emetics for his nausea, and oral balance gel for his dry mouth. K^+ supplements were given and mexilitine added to amiodarone to try and minimize the risk of VT.

Jim, his wife, and three children were involved in the discussion about planning for future appropriate care at this stage of his illness leading to:

- Deactivation of the ICD with medication to try to minimize further VT.
- Establishing that Jim's preferred place of care was at home.
- An understanding and agreement that resuscitation would be futile and not in Jim's best interests.

He was therefore discharged with the following support in place:

- General practitioner (GP), HF nurse specialist, district nurse, and community palliative care support.

• Anticipatory care plan including Jim's wishes and a plan in place for possible medical complications such as what to do in the event of further VT.

Jim died at home, in comfort and surrounded by his family. No further hospital admissions were needed. Bereavement support was provided for the family following his death.

References

1 Cleland JG, Khand A, Clark A (2001) The heart failure epidemic: exactly how big is it? *Eur Heart J* **22**, 623–6.
2 McMurray JJ, Stewart S (2000) Epidemiology, aetiology, and prognosis of heart failure. *Heart* **83**, 596–602.
3 Jaarsma T, Beattie JM, Ryder M (2009) Palliative care in heart failure: a position statement from the palliative care workshop of the Heart Failure Association of the European Society of Cardiology. *Eur J Heart Failure* **11**, 433–43.
4 Goodlin SJ, Hauptman PJ, Arnold R et al. (2004) Consensus statement: palliative and supportive care in advanced heart failure. *J Cardiac Failure* **10**, 200–9.
5 Formiga F, López-Soto A, Navarro M, Riera-Mestre A, Bosch X, Pujol R (2008) Hospital deaths of people aged 90 and over: end-of-life palliative care management. *Gerontology* **54**, 148–52.
6 Formiga F, Chivite D, Ortega C, Casas S, Ramón JM, Pujol R (2004) End-of-life preferences in elderly patients admitted for heart failure. *Q J Med* **97**, 803–8.
7 Dickstein K, Cohen-Solal A, Filippatos G et al. (2008) ESC guidelines for the diagnosis and treatment of acute and chronic heart failure. The Task Force for the Diagnosis and Treatment of Acute and Chronic Heart Failure 2008 of the European Society of Cardiology. Developed in collaboration with the Heart Failure Association of the ESC (HFA) and endorsed by the European Society of Intensive Care Medicine (ESICM). *Eur J Heart Failure* **10**, 933–89.
8 Davies E, Higginson IJ (eds) (2004) *Better palliative care for older people.* World Health Organization, Geneva (http://www.euro.who.int/__data/assets/pdf_file/0009/98235/E82933.pdf).
9 Gardiner C, Cobb M, Gott M, Ingleton C (2011) Barriers to providing palliative care for older people in acute hospitals. *Age Ageing* **40**, 233–8.
10 Murray SA, Boyd K, Sheikh A (2005) Palliative care in chronic illness. We need to move from prognostic paralysis to active total care. *BMJ* **330**, 611–12.
11 Stewart S, McMurray JJV (2002) Palliative care for heart failure. *BMJ* **325**, 915–16

The physiology of patients with HF: the origin of symptoms and rationale for treatment

Definition and classification of HF

HF is defined as a syndrome where patients demonstrate symptoms and signs of HF such as dyspnoea, fatigue, pulmonary congestion, and peripheral oedema in the context of objective evidence of structural and/or functional cardiac abnormalities at rest.[1]

Currently recommended terms to describe HF presentations are:[1]

- 'New onset' denoting the first presentation of HF.
- 'Transient' indicating recurrent or episodic HF perhaps secondary to ischaemia or myocarditis.
- 'Chronic' where the syndrome is persistent, progressive, and prone to decompensation.

Chronic HF is often further classified by functional status (Table 2.1).

A distinction is made between those with reduced ejection fraction and those with preserved ejection fraction. The latter often comprises patients with diastolic HF, right HF, and valvular heart disease. Patients with HF and preserved ejection fraction represent up to 50% of all patients with HF and have a similar prognosis to those with HF and reduced ejection fraction.

Table 2.1 NYHA functional classification

NYHA I	No limitation of ordinary physical activity
NYHA II	Slight limitation of ordinary physical activity by dyspnoea, fatigue or palpitation
NYHA III	Marked limitation of less than ordinary physical activity by dyspnoea, fatigue or palpitation
NYHA IV	Symptomatic at rest with increased discomfort with any physical activity

Reprinted from The Criteria Committee of the New York Heart Association, Nomenclature and Criteria for Diagnosis of Diseases of the Heart and Great Vessels, 9th edition, Wolters Kluwer Health, 1994, pp. 253–256, with permission of Lippincott Williams & Wilkins.

Aetiology of HF

HF is the clinical consequence of myocardial damage and dysfunction. Coronary artery disease is the most common cause in the Western world. Other causes are listed in Box 2.1.

Box 2.1 The aetiology of chronic HF

- Coronary artery disease.
- Valvular heart disease.
- Hypertension.
- Adult congenital heart disease.
- Alcohol excess.
- Tachyarrhythmia.
- Cardiomyopathies: including dilated, hypertrophic, restrictive, and peripartum.
- Infiltrative disease: including amyloid, sarcoid, and haemochromatosis.
- Pericardial disease.
- Recreational drugs, e.g. cocaine.
- Cardiotoxic drugs, e.g. anthracyclines and trastuzumab.
- Infections, e.g. viral myocarditis, Chagas disease, and human immunodeficiency virus (HIV).
- Nutritional deficiency, e.g. thiamine and beriberi.
- High-output failure, e.g. anaemia, thyrotoxicosis, and Paget's disease.

Pathophysiology of HF

Cardiac dysfunction, irrespective of aetiology, effects a reduction in stroke volume and a consequent fall in cardiac output. This triggers numerous compensatory haemodynamic, neurohumoral, and structural responses. Whilst initially effective in restoring and maintaining cardiac output, over time these responses are maladaptive and contribute to adverse ventricular remodelling and a further decline in cardiac function.

Haemodynamic response

- Increased left ventricular end-diastolic volume.
- Increased pulmonary capillary wedge pressure.

The reduction in stroke volume increases the volume of blood remaining in the left ventricle after myocardial contraction. This augments left ventricular end-diastolic volume resulting in ventricular dilatation and initiation of the Frank–Starling mechanism. 'Starling's law' dictates that as muscle fibre stretch increases so does the force of muscle contraction. However, this is only true up to a point, after which further muscle fibre stretch does not result in increased myocardial contraction (Fig. 2.1).

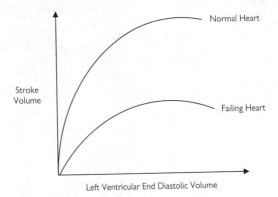

Fig. 2.1. The Frank–Starling mechanism.

Autonomic nervous system response

- Increased sympathetic adrenergic activity.
- Reduced vagal activity to heart.

Baroreceptors detecting a fall in cardiac output activate the sympathetic nervous system, stimulating an increase in circulating catecholamines. The effect on cardiac function is both chronotropic and inotropic with elevation of heart rate and increased force of myocardial contraction. Peripheral vasoconstriction in response to sympathetic activation increases venous return to the heart which augments preload and therefore contractility by Starling's law. However, peripheral vasoconstriction also increases afterload which has the effect of increasing myocardial work and oxygen demand.

Hormonal responses

- Activation of renin–angiotensin–aldosterone system (RAAS).
- Release of antidiuretic hormone.
- Release of natriuretic peptides.

The RAAS is activated by diminished renal perfusion secondary to a reduction in cardiac output (Fig. 2.2). This promotes the production of angiotensin II, a potent vasoconstrictor. The effect is an increase in preload which by Starling's law increases myocardial contractility. Angiotensin II also stimulates the production of aldosterone by the adrenal glands, which serves to increase circulating blood volume by the retention of sodium and water. Whilst beneficially increasing preload in the acute setting, chronically this process is deleterious to cardiac function and promotes peripheral and pulmonary oedema. Activation of the RAAS also contributes to adverse ventricular remodelling by inducing:

- Myocyte hypertrophy.
- Myocyte fibrosis.
- Myocyte apoptosis.

Natriuretic peptides are secreted in response to atrial and ventricular stretch secondary to elevated left ventricular end-diastolic pressure. These promote vasodilation and the loss of sodium and water but are insufficient to counteract the negative effects of RAAS and sympathetic nervous system activation.

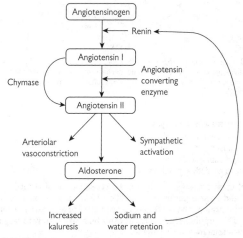

Fig. 2.2 The RAAS. Reproduced from Gardner, McDonagh and Walker, *Heart Failure*, 2007, p. 13 with permission of Oxford University Press.

Structural response
- Dilatation of damaged myocardium.
- Hypertrophy of unaffected myocytes.
- Fibrosis of necrotic myocardium.

The various haemodynamic and neurohumoral responses to the failing heart instigate structural changes within the myocardium referred to collectively as adverse ventricular remodelling. This process promotes a further decline in cardiac function and the development of a vicious cycle of progressive HF (Fig. 2.3).

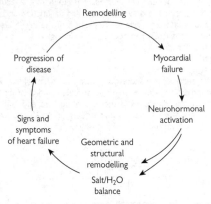

Fig. 2.3 Vicious cycle of progressive HF. Reproduced from *Heart*, Christian G Brilla, Renin-angiotensin system mediated mechanisms: cardioreparation and cardioprotection, Volume 84, Suppl 1: i18–i19, 2000 with permission from BMJ Publishing Group Ltd.

Skeletal muscle changes
- Muscle fibre fibrosis and atrophy.
- Intracellular lipid deposition.
- Reduced capillary density.
- Reduced oxidative metabolism.

Skeletal muscle changes in HF are the consequence of reduced cardiac output and muscle perfusion in addition to general deconditioning and deficient nutrition. The latter may be secondary to anorexia and impaired intestinal absorption. These changes contribute significantly to fatigue and exercise intolerance in HF patients.

Symptoms of HF (see 📖 Chapters 9 and 10)

The predominant symptoms of chronic HF are:
- Dyspnoea.
- Oedema.
- Fatigue.
- Pain.

Dyspnoea

Dyspnoea is the most common symptom of chronic HF and may be debilitating both in terms of poor exercise tolerance and psychological distress. The underlying pathophysiology is complex and not fully understood but probably involves:
- Elevation of pulmonary capillary wedge pressure with transudation of fluid into the lungs.
- Perfusion–ventilation mismatch within the lungs.
- Reduction in pulmonary compliance.
- Augmentation of chemoreceptor sensitivity.
- Skeletal muscle myopathy.

Importantly dyspnoea is not only a consequence of pulmonary oedema but often persists once the patient is euvolaemic. Dyspnoea in HF may be exacerbated by numerous concomitant related pathologies which are important to identify:
- Respiratory tract infection.
- Pleural effusion.
- Pulmonary embolism.
- Bronchial neoplasm.
- Atrial fibrillation.
- Anaemia.

Oedema

This is a common clinical feature in HF and can be particularly distressing during the later stages of the disease. Compensatory neurohumoral mechanisms in HF promote an increase in plasma volume and the consequent increase in capillary hydrostatic pressure drives fluid exudation. Gravitational forces contribute, so oedema is most often peripheral, at the ankles, in ambulant patients and sacral in those confined to bed. Pleural effusions and ascites may also develop. Chronic peripheral oedema may be painful and initiate skin breakdown, blistering, and infection. Worsening oedema may represent deteriorating cardiac function and progressive fluid retention, but other factors should be considered:
- Poor compliance with fluid restriction and medical therapy.
- Renal insufficiency.
- Hepatic insufficiency.
- Cellulitis.
- Deep-vein thrombosis.

Fatigue

Fatigue is a major manifestation of chronic HF, and most often the cause is multifactorial:

- Disrupted sleep due to orthopnoea, paroxysmal nocturnal dyspnoea, and central and/or obstructive sleep apnoea.
- Periodic breathing secondary to augmented chemosensitivity.
- Poor nutrition due to reduced appetite or malabsorption secondary to gastrointestinal oedema.
- Anaemia secondary to chronic disease or antiplatelet or anticoagulant therapy.
- Beta-blockers.
- Hypokalaemia secondary to diuretic therapy.
- Depression.

Pain

Pain is a common symptom, particularly in advanced HF. It is again multi-factorial often secondary to:

- Angina.
- Gastrointestinal congestion.
- Gross oedema.
- Gout secondary to diuretic therapy.
- Immobility.
- Psychological distress.

Treatment of HF

The management of HF comprises both pharmacological and non-pharmacological therapies including implantable devices and surgical interventions. The primary objectives of treatment in HF are to:

- Alleviate symptoms and improve quality of life.
- Avoid hospital admission.
- Prevent disease progression.
- Reduce mortality.

Diuretics

Diuretic therapy is essential in the management of symptomatic pulmonary and peripheral congestion and a recent Cochrane analysis presented trial evidence of both morbidity and mortality benefits.[2]

Loop and thiazide diuretics exert their effects on the loop of Henle and the distal tubule, respectively, promoting excretion of sodium and water. First-line diuretic therapy is a loop diuretic such as furosemide or bumetanide. Cautious dose titration is imperative to avoid excessive volume depletion and pre-renal failure. Higher doses of diuretics are often required in the context of more significant HF or if there is co-existing renal impairment. Thiazides such as bendroflumethiazide and metolazone may be used in conjunction with loop diuretics in resistant oedema. Hospital admission for intravenous diuretics is often necessary if absorption of oral medication becomes compromised by gastrointestinal oedema.

The objective is to prescribe the minimum diuretics required to achieve and maintain euvolaemia. Table 2.2 presents typical dose titration regimes. Importantly, when prescribing diuretics in HF patients should be educated with regards to complying with fluid restriction and monitoring weight gain. Some patients may even tailor their own diuretic dosage in accordance with weight gain or loss.

Table 2.2 Diuretics—drugs and dosing

Class	Diuretic	Starting dose	Common titrated doses	Concomitant therapy
Loop	Furosemide	40mg	80mg bd or 120mg bd	Alone or + thiazide
Loop	Bumetanide	1mg	2mg bd or 3mg bd	Alone or + thiazide
Thiazide	Bendroflu-methiazide	2.5mg	2.5mg weekly or 2 or 3 × weekly	Loop diuretic
Thiazide	Metolazone	2.5mg	2.5mg weekly or 2 or 3 × weekly	Loop diuretic

bd, twice a day.

Adverse effects from diuretic therapy are common and should be actively considered and monitored as appropriate:

- Hypokalaemia ± arrhythmia.
- Hyponatraemia.
- Intravascular volume depletion and pre-renal failure.
- Muscle cramps.
- Urinary frequency.
- Incontinence.
- Hyperuricaemia and gout.
- Glucose intolerance (thiazides).

ACE inhibitors

ACE inhibitors are the first-line medical therapy in all patients with HF irrespective of NYHA class. Large randomized double-blind placebo-controlled trials have irrefutably demonstrated their beneficial effects in terms of:[3–5]

- Improving ventricular function.
- Enhancing patient well-being.
- Reducing hospital admissions.
- Increasing survival.

ACE inhibitors inhibit the RAAS by reducing the production of angiotensin II and slowing the breakdown of bradykinin (Fig. 2.4). These actions promote vasodilation and a consequent reduction in afterload and myocardial work. Furthermore, diminishing downstream production of aldosterone beneficially reduces sodium and water retention. Inhibiting the RAAS may also ameliorate adverse ventricular remodelling.

Table 2.3 depicts commonly used ACE inhibitors and their recommended starting and target doses. Starting therapy at a low dose is recommended with up-titration weekly or fortnightly dependent on blood pressure, symptomatic hypotension and renal function.

Table 2.3 RAAS inhibition in HF—drugs and dosing

Class	Drug	Starting dose	Target dose
ACE inhibitor	Captopril	6.25mg	50mg tds
ACE inhibitor	Enalapril	2.5mg	20mg bd
ACE inhibitor	Lisinopril	5mg	40mg od
ACE inhibitor	Ramipril	2.5mg	5mg bd
Angiotensin II receptor antagonist	Candesartan	4mg	32mg od
Angiotensin II receptor antagonist	Losartan	25mg	100mg od

(Continued)

Table 2.3 (cont'd.)

Class	Drug	Starting dose	Target dose
Angiotensin II receptor antagonist	Valsartan	40mg	160mg bd
Aldosterone antagonist	Spironolactone	25mg	50mg od
Aldosterone antagonist	Eplerenone	25mg	50mg od

tds, three times a day; od, once a day.

The major adverse effects of ACE inhibition are hypotension and renal impairment. Nocturnal dosing may alleviate symptomatic hypotension. A degree of deterioration in renal function is considered acceptable but the ACE inhibitor should be withdrawn if creatinine rises more than 50% above baseline or reaches 266µmol/L.[1]

Contraindications to the introduction of an ACE inhibitor are:
• Hyperkalaemia.
• Bilateral renal artery stenosis.
• Previous ACE inhibitor-induced cough (5–10%).
• Previous ACE inhibitor-induced angio-oedema.
• Severe renal impairment without renal replacement therapy.
• Pregnancy.
• Significant symptomatic hypotension with systolic blood pressure (BP) < 90mmHg.
• Severe aortic stenosis.

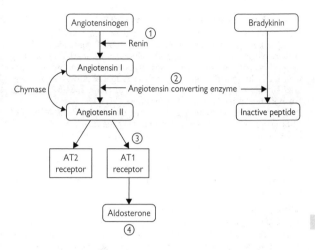

1. Renin inhibitor
2. ACE inhibitor
3. Angiotensin receptor antagonist
4. Aldosterone antagonist

Fig. 2.4 The sites of action of antagonists of the RAAS. Reproduced from Gardner, McDonagh and Walker, *Heart Failure*, 2007, p. 427 with permission of Oxford University Press.

Angiotensin II receptor antagonists (ARBs)

ACE inhibitors do not completely prevent the production of angiotensin II (Fig. 2.4). Angiotensin II receptor antagonists (ARBs) provide a different pharmacological mechanism of RAAS blockade. By specifically blocking the AT1 receptor an ARB effects vasodilation, sodium and water excretion, and reduced antidiuretic hormone secretion. As ARBs do not inhibit bradykinin breakdown, adverse effects such as cough and angio-oedema are much less likely than with ACE inhibitors.

Large randomized controlled trials have demonstrated the efficacy of ARBs in improving morbidity and mortality in patients with HF.[6–9] An ARB is therefore an appropriate alternative therapy for patients intolerant of ACE inhibitors, for example due to cough.[1] There is also evidence of a morbidity and mortality benefit when an ARB is prescribed in addition to otherwise maximal therapy with an ACE inhibitor and beta-blocker.[8] Table 2.3 depicts commonly utilized ARBs and their recommended starting and target doses.

Aldosterone antagonists

It is well recognized that the suppression of aldosterone production by ACE inhibitors and ARBs is only transient, since mechanisms other than the RAAS contribute to aldosterone release. Aldosterone antagonists such as spironolactone and eplerenone bind to mineralocorticoid receptors, reducing sodium and water retention and inhibiting adverse ventricular remodelling.

Clinical trial evidence supports the use of aldosterone antagonists in patients with NYHA II–IV HF and patients with reduced left ventricular ejection fraction (LVEF) following myocardial infarction (MI).[10–12] An ACE inhibitor or ARB in addition to a beta-blocker should be initiated in the first instance and an aldosterone antagonist added if symptoms persist and it is likely to be tolerated in terms of blood pressure, renal function, and hyperkalaemia. Table 2.3 depicts the recommended starting and target doses of spironolactone and eplerenone.

The most important adverse effect of aldosterone antagonists is hyperkalaemia and this should be actively monitored. Spironolactone is a non-selective aldosterone antagonist and as such binds to androgen and progesterone receptors and may induce painful gynaecomastia. Eplerenone is selective for the mineralocorticoid receptor and is therefore a useful alternative.

Beta-blockers

Beta-blockers counteract the deleterious effects of sympathetic nervous system activation in HF. A large body of evidence has unequivocally demonstrated their favourable effects:[13–16]
- Improving ventricular function.
- Enhancing patient well-being.
- Reducing hospital admissions.
- Increasing survival.

Table 2.4 presents the beta-blockers with proven efficacy in HF and their recommended starting and target doses.

Beta-blocker therapy is indicated in all patients with NYHA II–IV HF. It should be introduced at a low dose and titrated cautiously, every 1–2 weeks, as BP, heart rate, and clinical symptoms and signs of fluid retention permit.

Contraindications to commencing beta-blocker therapy are:

- Second- or third-degree heart block without permanent pacemaker implantation.
- Decompensated HF.
- Critical peripheral vascular disease.
- Significant symptomatic hypotension with systolic BP < 90mmHg.
- Severe airflow obstruction with reversibility.

Table 2.4 Beta-blockers in HF—drugs and dosing

Drug	Starting dose	Target dose
Bisoprolol	1.25mg	10mg od
Carvedilol	3.125mg	25mg bd*
Metoprolol XL	12.5/25mg	200mg od
Nebivolol	1.25mg	10mg od

*Patients > 85kg target dose 50mg bd

Digoxin

Digoxin, a cardiac glycoside, is a positive inotrope with additional properties that slow conduction across the AV node. The Digitalis Investigation Group (DIG) trial demonstrated that in severe refractory HF the addition of digoxin improved symptoms and reduced hospital admissions but did not affect mortality.[17] Correspondingly the addition of digoxin is recommended in chronic HF only where symptoms persist despite maximal tolerated therapy with an ACE inhibitor or ARB, a beta-blocker, and an aldosterone antagonist.[1] Digoxin is also indicated for ventricular rate control in HF patients with concomitant atrial fibrillation in whom a beta-blocker is either insufficient or inappropriate.

Digoxin therapy has several potential undesirable effects which should be considered when prescribing:

- Narrow therapeutic window with risk of toxicity.
- Increased cardiac toxicity in context of hypokalaemia.
- Dose adjustment requirement in renal impairment.
- Drug interactions with increased plasma concentration of digoxin with:
  - amiodarone
  - propafenone and quinidine
  - spironolactone.
- Pro-arrhythmic.
- Multiple side-effects.

Hydralazine and nitrates

Hydralazine is an arteriolar dilator which exerts its beneficial effect on cardiac output by reducing afterload. Nitrates are venodilators at low doses but induce arterial dilatation at higher doses. The combination of hydralazine and isosorbide dinitrate (H-ISDN) has been demonstrated to improve morbidity and mortality in HF but to a lesser extent than ACE inhibition.[18] African-American patients in particular may have a more significant mortality benefit from H-ISDN therapy.[19]

H-ISDN is primarily recommended where neither an ACE inhibitor nor ARB are tolerated. It may also be indicated in patients who remain symptomatic despite otherwise maximal medical therapy including an ACE inhibitor or ARB.[1] Contraindications to use include significant renal dysfunction and hypotension.

ICDs

Ventricular arrhythmia is common in HF and up to 50% of HF deaths are attributable to sudden cardiac death. It has been demonstrated that ICDs reduce mortality in otherwise optimally treated patients with ischaemic or non-ischaemic HF.[20,21] As such, ICD implantation is recommended for primary or secondary prevention of sudden cardiac death in otherwise optimally treated HF patients as follows:[1]

- Primary prevention:
  - NYHA II–III HF at least 40 days post-MI with LVEF ≤ 35%, with expectation of survival > 1 year.
  - Non-ischaemic NYHA II–III HF with LVEF ≤ 35% with expectation of survival > 1 year.
- Secondary prevention:
  - Survivors of ventricular fibrillation.
  - Haemodynamically unstable VT with expectation of survival > 1 year.

CRT

CRT is aimed at reducing the interventricular dyssynchrony and atrioventricular conduction delay that occur in HF. A CRT pacemaker (CRTP) requires pacing leads in the right atrium (except in the context of permanent atrial fibrillation), right ventricle, and coronary sinus (to pace the left ventricular free wall) and it may be combined with an internal cardiac defibrillator (CRTD). CRTP in patients with NYHA III–IV HF despite otherwise optimal medical therapy has been demonstrated in large randomized controlled trials to:[22,23]

- Increase survival.
- Improve symptoms and exercise tolerance.
- Reduce hospital admissions.

Consideration of CRTP is currently recommended in patients with chronic HF who fulfil all of the following criteria:[1]

- NYHA III–IV HF despite optimal medical therapy with ACE inhibitor or ARB, beta-blocker, and aldosterone antagonist.
- Reduced LVEF (≤ 35%).
- QRS prolongation on electrocardiogram (ECG) (QRS width ≥ 120ms).

CRTD rather than CRTP is indicated in HF patients who also fulfil the criteria for an ICD.[1]

Surgical intervention

Surgical interventions in HF include revascularization, left ventricular reconstruction surgery, mitral valve surgery, mechanical cardiac support, and cardiac transplant and are summarized in Fig. 2.5.

Surgical revascularization, or indeed percutaneous coronary intervention, in ischaemic HF may be appropriate in certain circumstances dependent on symptoms, coronary anatomy, extent of myocardial viability comorbidities, and procedural risk. Revascularization in HF, however, remains controversial, with the recent STICH I trial demonstrating no significant difference in all-cause mortality between coronary artery bypass surgery plus optimal medical therapy as compared with optimal medical therapy alone in patients with a median LVEF of 28%.[24]

Significant functional mitral regurgitation (MR) is common in chronic HF due to increased left ventricular sphericity which widens the interpapillary angle and results in tethering of the mitral valve leaflets. Mitral valve annular dilatation also contributes. Mitral valve repair, most commonly with an annular ring, improves symptoms. Mitral valve replacement is not routinely recommended for functional MR in chronic HF as the altered left ventricular geometry post-operatively may have a detrimental effect on cardiac function.

Recent technological advances have permitted the use of mechanical cardiac support including ventricular assist devices and artificial hearts in some HF patients in specific circumstances. Currently the most common indication for a ventricular assist device is as a bridge to cardiac transplantation. Whilst there is some evidence to support mechanical cardiac support as destination therapy in patients ineligible for transplantation, experience of this limited.[25]

Cardiac transplantation is an accepted treatment for patients with advanced HF who remain symptomatic despite optimal HF therapies. Transplantation affords improved quality of life and survival in appropriately selected recipients. It does, however, have its own significant associated morbidity and mortality and as such is only a realistic option for a small percentage of patients. For most, the ceiling of therapy is reached well before cardiac transplantation.

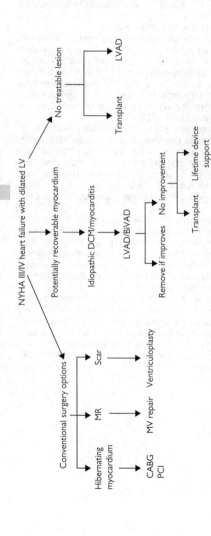

Fig. 2.5 Surgical options in HF (LV, left ventricle; CABG, coronary artery bypass graft; PCI, percutaneous coronary intervention; MV, mitral valve; LVAD, left ventricular assist device; BiVAD, biventricular assist device; DCM, dilated cardiomyopathy). Reproduced from Gardner, McDonagh and Walker, *Heart Failure*, 2007, p. 105 with permission of Oxford University Press.

References

1 Dickstein K, Cohen-Solal A, Filippatos G et al. (2008) ESC guidelines for the diagnosis and treatment of acute and chronic heart failure 2008: the Task Force for the Diagnosis and Treatment of Acute and Chronic Heart Failure 2008 of the European Society of Cardiology. Developed in collaboration with the Heart Failure Association of the ESC (HFA) and endorsed by the European Society of Intensive Care Medicine (ESICM). *Eur Heart J* **29**, 2388–42.

2 Faris R, Flather MD, Purcell H et al. (2006) Diuretics for heart failure. *Cochrane Database Syst Rev* 2006(1):CD003838.

3 [No authors listed] (1987) Effects of enalapril on mortality in severe congestive heart failure. Results of the Cooperative North Scandinavian Enalapril Survival Study (CONSENSUS). The CONSENSUS Trial Study Group. *N Engl J Med* **316**, 1429–35.

4 [No authors listed] (1991) Effect of enalapril on survival in patients with reduced left ventricular ejection fractions and congestive heart failure. The SOLVD Investigators. *N Engl J Med* **325**, 293–302.

5 Pfeffer MA, Braunwald E, Moye LA et al. (1992) Effect of captopril on mortality and morbidity in patients with left ventricular dysfunction after myocardial infarction. Results of the survival and ventricular enlargement trial. The SAVE Investigators. *N Engl J Med* **327**, 669–77.

6 Cohn JN, Tognoni G (2001) A randomized trial of the angiotensin-receptor blocker valsartan in chronic heart failure. *N Engl J Med* **345**, 1667–75.

7 Granger CB, McMurray JJ, Yusuf S et al. (2003) Effects of candesartan in patients with chronic heart failure and reduced left-ventricular systolic function intolerant to angiotensin-converting-enzyme inhibitors: the CHARM-Alternative trial. *Lancet* **362**, 772–6.

8 McMurray JJ, Ostergren J, Swedberg K et al. (2003) Effects of candesartan in patients with chronic heart failure and reduced left-ventricular systolic function taking angiotensin-converting-enzyme inhibitors: the CHARM-Added trial. *Lancet* **362**, 767–71.

9 Pitt B, Poole-Wilson PA, Segal R et al. (2000) Effect of losartan compared with captopril on mortality in patients with symptomatic heart failure: randomised trial – the Losartan Heart Failure Survival Study ELITE II. *Lancet* **355**, 1582–7.

10 Pitt B, Zannad F, Remme WJ et al. (1999) The effect of spironolactone on morbidity and mortality in patients with severe heart failure. Randomized Aldactone Evaluation Study Investigators. *N Engl J Med* **341**, 709–17.

11 Pitt B, Remme W, Zannad F et al. (2003) Eplerenone, a selective aldosterone blocker, in patients with left ventricular dysfunction after myocardial infarction. *N Engl J Med* **348**, 1309–21.

12 Zannad F, McMurray JJ, Krum H et al. (2011) Eplerenone in patients with systolic heart failure and mild symptoms. *N Engl J Med* **364**, 11–21.

13 [No authors listed] (1999) The Cardiac Insufficiency Bisoprolol Study II (CIBIS-II): a randomised trial. *Lancet* **353**, 9–13.

14 Dargie HJ (2001) Effect of carvedilol on outcome after myocardial infarction in patients with left-ventricular dysfunction: the CAPRICORN randomised trial. *Lancet* **357**, 1385–90.

15 [No authors listed] (1999) Effect of metoprolol CR/XL in chronic heart failure: Metoprolol CR/XL Randomised Intervention Trial in Congestive Heart Failure (MERIT-HF). *Lancet* **353**, 2001–7.

16 Packer M, Coats AJ, Fowler MB et al. (2001) Effect of carvedilol on survival in severe chronic heart failure. *N Engl J Med* **344**, 1651–8.

17 [No authors listed] (1997) The effect of digoxin on mortality and morbidity in patients with heart failure. The Digitalis Investigation Group. *N Engl J Med* **336**, 525–33.

18 Cohn JN, Johnson G, Ziesche S et al. (1991) A comparison of enalapril with hydralazine-isosorbide dinitrate in the treatment of chronic congestive heart failure. *N Engl J Med* **325**, 303–10.

19 Taylor AL, Ziesche S, Yancy C et al. (2004) Combination of isosorbide dinitrate and hydralazine in blacks with heart failure. *N Engl J Med* **351**, 2049–57.

20 Moss AJ, Zareba W, Hall WJ et al. (2002) Prophylactic implantation of a defibrillator in patients with myocardial infarction and reduced ejection fraction. *N Engl J Med* **346**, 877–83.

21 Bardy GH, Lee KL, Mark DB et al. (2005) Amiodarone or an implantable cardioverter-defibrillator for congestive heart failure. *N Engl J Med* **352**, 225–37.

22 Cleland JG, Daubert JC, Erdmann E et al. (2005) The effect of cardiac resynchronization on morbidity and mortality in heart failure. *N Engl J Med* **352**, 1539–49.

23 Bristow MR, Saxon LA, Boehmer J et al. (2004) Cardiac-resynchronization therapy with or without an implantable defibrillator in advanced chronic heart failure. *N Engl J Med* **350**, 2140–50.

24 Velazquez EJ, Lee KL, Deja MA et al. (2011) Coronary-artery bypass surgery in patients with left ventricular dysfunction. *N Engl J Med* **364**, 1607–16.

25 Rose EA, Gelijns AC, Moskowitz AJ et al. (2001) Long-term use of a left ventricular assist device for end-stage heart failure. *N Engl J Med* **345**, 1435–43.

Prognostication and disease trajectory

Introduction

While the prognosis for HF is well known to be poor, prognostication at any stage in HF has always been difficult. Indeed as the potential therapeutic strategies for HF have become more varied and complex, prognostication has become harder. The challenge surrounding prognostication is primarily related to the unpredictable illness trajectory (Fig. 3.1) compared with that of some types of cancer, particularly those with fewer treatment options such as lung cancer (Fig. 3.2). The type of illness trajectory in cancer allows for an element of planning by the medical teams and a time for preparation and adaptation for the patient and their family at the, usually, easy to recognize stage when the patient begins to deteriorate. This is in contrast to the chaotic illness trajectory followed by patients with HF.

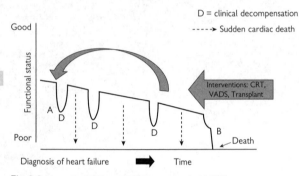

Fig. 3.1 Unpredictable illness trajectory associated with HF.*

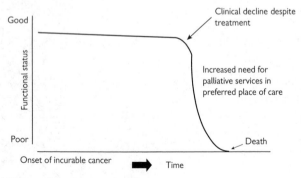

Fig. 3.2 Illness trajectory associated with some cancers.*

*Figs 3.1 and 3.2: Adapted from Joanne Lynn and David M. Adamson, Living Well at the End of Life: Adapting Health Care to Serious Chronic Illness in Old Age, 2003 with permission from the RAND Corporation, Santa Monica California, USA and Scott A. Murray et al., Illness Trajectories and Palliative Care, BMJ Vol. 330, No. 7498, pp. 1007–1011, copyright © 2005, with permission from the BMJ Publishing Group Ltd.

Difficulties due to an unpredictable trajectory (see Fig. 3.1)
- Patients have multiple episodes of clinical decompensation requiring hospitalization (points D in Fig. 3.1).
- Patients at these points are sick enough to die but can make a reasonable recovery back to their premorbid state and are discharged home.
- Methods to assess if a patient will die during that period of clinical decompensation are unreliable; it is difficult to know if a patient is at point A or point B. Stopping therapy at point A would mean that a patient would miss out on life between points A and B which may or may not be a reasonable quality of life.
- The incidence of sudden cardiac death increases as the LVEF falls.
- Some interventions such as CRT, ventricular assist devices (VADs), and cardiac transplantation can move the patient to the left of the graph or acutely to the right in some cases as each intervention has a mortality and morbidity of its own.
- Many patients are not suitable for these interventions, and for those who are there is no guarantee that they will be successful with regard to survival or symptomatic benefit; only 70% of patients will gain symptomatic benefit after CRT and these people cannot be predicted at the time of implant.

Scoring systems and prognostication

Improving prognostication and identifying patients early may allow for improvements in end of life care. Patients most in need of the palliative and supportive care strategies might be identified and plans put in place for good end of life care individualized to patients' needs.

Within HF there are a number of single-item predictors of poor prognosis:

- NYHA class.
- Six-minute walk test.
- Maximal oxygen consumption (VO2max).
- Prolonged QRS duration.
- Natriuretic peptides such as brain natriuretic peptide (BNP) and N-terminal proBNP.[1–5]

However, no single factor is a perfect predictor of prognosis, and as such multivariate models have been developed. A comprehensive discussion is beyond the scope of this chapter, but the two most common models include the HF Survival Score (HFSS)—used mainly to assess suitability for cardiac transplantation—and the Seattle HF Score (SHFS).[6,7] These models include a variety of factors such as:

- Age.
- Aetiology of HF.
- LVEF.
- NYHA class.
- QRS duration, heart rate, mean arterial pressure.
- Peak VO$_2$.
- Diuretic dose.
- Haemoglobin, uric acid, serum creatinine, and serum sodium.

However neither model includes biochemical markers of prognosis and they do not take into account the impact of comorbidities. These models attempt to form scoring mechanisms that could be used to rank patients into those most in need of palliative care.

Applying these scores to an individual, however, can be difficult. In practice, clinical experience and careful assessment of the patient in light of the course that the disease is taking is often the most appropriate approach. The Gold Standards Framework (GSF)[8] proposes the GSF Prognostic Indicator guidance as a tool to assist the generalist clinician to identify patients approaching the end stage of their disease (Box 3.1). The guidance acts to provide 'triggers' for health care professionals to make supportive measures for end of life care a priority.

Haga *et al.*[9] recently demonstrated that neither the GSF nor the SHF score accurately predicted which patients were in their last year of life. Distinct from formal scoring systems there are often more specific clinical features which can indicate a decline in status and a poor prognosis which could act as 'triggers' for discussion and review of a patient's palliative care needs (Box 3.2).

Box 3.1 Triggers for supportive/palliative care[8]

- The surprise question: Would you be surprised if this patient were to die in 6–12 months?
- Patient choice/need: The patient with advanced disease makes a choice for comfort care only, e.g. refusing cardiac transplant or VAD.
- Disease-specific indicators requiring at least two of the following indicators:
  - NYHA III or IV HF
  - Patient felt to be in last year of life by main care team
  - Repeated hospital admissions with HF.
- Distressing physical or psychological symptoms despite optimally tolerated therapy.

Box 3.2 Triggers[1,5,10,11]

- Progressive renal dysfunction.
- 5% non-fluid-related weight loss resulting in cardiac cachexia.
- Escalating diuretic dose requirements.
- Recurrent admissions with HF within 6-month period despite optimally tolerated HF therapy.
- IV diuretic ± IV inotrope dependence or increase in frequency of need with no further therapeutic strategy.
- Deteriorating quality of life despite optimally tolerated HF therapy.
- Occurrence of malignant arrhythmias or increase in discharges from ICD.
- Albumin < 2.5g/dL.
- Ejection fraction (EF) < 20%.
- Prior CPR.
- Inability to tolerate optimal dose, or any, cardiac medication.
- Persistent hyponatraemia.

The relevance of scoring systems in the assessment of palliative care needs

The need for formal scoring systems, rather than clinical recognition of triggers in the context of a patient's overall progress, is more important if we follow a model of care that discharges the HF patient from cardiology and completely transfers the care to palliative care when the patient reaches a designated stage of disease (Fig. 3.3).

However, this model is based on the outdated and unhelpful school of thought that palliative care is only for patients who have reached the terminal phase of their illness. If palliative care needs and specialist palliative care referral are only thought of once clinicians feel certain that a patient is in the last few weeks or months of life, then there will be 'prognostic paralysis' (see 📖 Chapter 1) whereby these issues remain unaddressed.

Therefore the inadequacy of current scoring systems is irrelevant to the issue of whether patients access palliative care support, whether from generalist or specialist providers.

Access to palliative care should be based on the patient's problems rather than prognosis.[12] Although, in practice, the two are often synonymous, it does allow that, on occasion, a patient who has required palliative care may improve if they respond to therapy. In this case, the problems will resolve and palliative needs will lessen. If specialist services have been involved, the patient can be discharged and re-referred later if necessary.

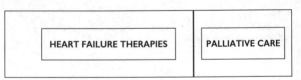

HEART FAILURE THERAPIES   **PALLIATIVE CARE**

Fig. 3.3 Box model of palliative care.

Escaping 'prognostic paralysis'

The 'phases' of HF

Boyd *et al.*[13] following a longitudinal study, describe three phases of HF: chronic disease management; supportive and palliative care; dying. They describe the following characteristics and suggest that a transition in performance status—or again the 'sentinel' hospital admission—should herald a trigger for reassessment and consideration of a palliative care approach.

- Phase 1. Chronic disease management: NYHA I–II, Karnofsky Performance Status (KPS) 80–100%.
- Phase 2. Supportive and palliative care: NYHA III–IV, KPS 50–70%.
- Phase 3. Dying: NYHA IV or KPS < 50%.

Problem-based approach to palliative care—not a prognosis-based approach

With this approach:

- Palliative care and cardiology work collaboratively and in parallel (Fig. 3.4).
- Symptom needs of the patient can continuously be assessed.
- Trigger points (Box 3.2) would stimulate review and assessment of the palliative needs of the patient and family thorough the patient's journey and into bereavement.
- Palliative care focuses on a holistic approach to symptom management and is part of the umbrella which incorporates supportive care, end of life care, and bereavement care.
- If a patient's problems resolve, and their disease trajectory appears to move to the left, then this approach still allows for palliative care to be provided in a timely fashion when needed.

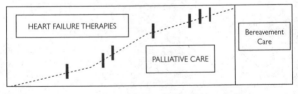

Fig. 3.4 Box model of palliative care and cardiology. Bold vertical lines represent trigger points.

A 'problem-based' approach with 'triggers' to signal the need for palliative care seems the best approach to management of patients with advanced HF. The broken line in Fig. 3.4 between cardiology and palliative care management signifies the ability to provide this problem-based approach to a patient's symptom needs and as such allows for cardiology and palliative care to work in parallel, using a collaborative approach to patient care for those with end-stage HF.

This type of approach:

- Is flexible enough to allow for timely access to generalist palliative care provided by the local team when needed despite the unpredictable illness trajectory that many of these patients will follow.
- It allows referral, if needed, to specialist palliative care for persistent or complex problems to occur seamlessly.
- Focuses on the management of problems as they arise. Attempting to address the issue by focusing on prognostication will always be difficult and is likely to present a barrier preventing access to appropriate palliative assessment and care.

References

1 Adler ED, Goldfinger JZ, Kalman J, Park ME, Meier DE (2009) Palliative care in the treatment of advanced heart failure. *Circulation* **120**, 2597–606.

2 Mancini DM, Eisen H, Kussmaul W, Mull R, Edmunds LH Jr, Wilson JR (1991) Value of peak exercise oxygen consumption for optimal timing of cardiac transplantation in ambulatory patients with heart failure. *Circulation* **83**, 778–86.

3 Metra M, Nodari S, Parrinello G et al. (2007) The role of plasma biomarkers in acute heart failure. Serial changes and independent prognostic value of NT-proBNP and cardiac troponin-T. *Eur J Heart Failure* **9**, 776–86.

4 Rothenburger M, Wichter T, Schmid C et al. (2004) Amino terminal pro type B natriuretic peptide as a predictive and prognostic marker in patients with chronic heart failure. *J Heart Lung Transplant* **23**, 1189–97.

5 Jaarsma T, Beattie JM, Ryder M (2009) Palliative care in heart failure: a position statement from the palliative care workshop of the Heart Failure Association of the European Society of Cardiology. *Eur J Heart Failure* **11**, 433–43.

6 Koelling TM, Joseph S, Aaronson KD (2004) Heart failure survival score continues to predict clinical outcomes in patients with heart failure receiving beta-blockers. *J Heart Lung Transplant* **23**, 1414–22.

7 Levy WC, Mozaffarian D, Linker DT et al. (2006) The Seattle Heart Failure Model: prediction of survival in heart failure. *Circulation* **113**, 1424–33.

8 The GSF prognostic indicator guidance. *End of Life Care* (2010) **4**(1).

9 Haga KK, Denvir MA, Reid J et al. (2011) Identifying patients with chronic heart failure who may benefit from palliative care: a comparison of the Gold Standards Framework with a clinical prognostic mode. *BMJ Support Palliat Care* **1**, A8.

10 Metra M, Ponikowski P, Dickstein K et al. (2007) Heart Failure Association of the European Society of Cardiology. Advanced chronic heart failure: a position statement from the Study Group on Advanced Heart Failure of the Heart Failure Association of the European Society of Cardiology. *Eur J Heart Failure* **9**, 684–94.

11 Pocock SJ, McMurray JJ, Dobson J et al. on behalf of the CHARM Investigators (2008) Weight loss and mortality risk in patients with chronic heart failure in the candesartan in heart failure: assessment of reduction in mortality and morbidity (CHARM) programme. *Eur Heart J* **29**, 2641–50.

12 Johnson MJ, Gadoud A (2011) Palliative care for people with chronic heart failure: when is it time? *J Palliat Care* **27**, 137–42.

13 Boyd KJ, Worth A, Kendall M et al. (2009) Making sure services deliver for people with advanced heart failure: a longitudinal qualitative study of patients, family carers, and health professionals. *Palliat Med* **23**, 767–76.

Communication in HF

Introduction

As prevalence of and available treatments for HF have increased, so has the need for clear and timely communication. Patients and their health care team need to discuss the nature and course of HF, prognosis, treatment options, and patient preferences for end of life care. The latter aspect has been highlighted in the recent GMC guidance.[1]

It is important that patients are given the opportunity to:

- Be better informed.
- Plan their lives.
- Take a more active role in the management of their illness.
- Be more likely to comply with best management.

Repeated studies over the past decade have highlighted that patients and their caregivers lack information and insight with regard to their diagnosis, management, and stage of illness.

What needs to be communicated?

Before anything is said, an assessment of what information a patient and their caregiver wishes to have and which areas of discussion are welcomed is paramount. The way in which important issues are discussed, or whether they are discussed at all, varies. It is important that communication is tailored to the individual. For some, the avoidance of bad news may be a long-term coping strategy that has served them well in the past. For whatever reason, this wish needs to be explored and usually respected if that is the patient's preferred approach.

Diagnosis and implications

- Explanation about the nature of the condition, and possible causes.
- Underlying physical changes and associated symptoms.
- Possible impact of symptoms on daily life.
- Terminology: the term 'heart failure' may not be familiar to or understood by patients.

Management

- Therapeutic options available, including pharmacological and non-drug therapies such as devices or transplant, and potential burdens or side-effects of treatment.
- Education regarding medication and treatment.
- Patient's and caregiver's information needs and psychosocial concerns.
- Information and support on how to achieve as good a quality of life as possible.

Prognosis

- A difficult but highly important aspect of communication in HF. If handled well it enables patients and their families to make plans and set priorities.
- Many patients with HF are ready for, and would welcome, information regarding prognosis; however, they may not ask about prognosis unprompted.
- Maintaining hope is important whilst recognizing that many patients with advanced disease can be overly optimistic about their prognosis.

Advance care planning (see 📖 Chapter 8)

Advance care planning (ACP) is a process of discussion between an individual, their care providers, and often those close to them, about future care:

- ACP provides a framework for patients to inform decision-making should they lose capacity.[2]
- ACP includes the documentation of conversations that happen as a part of good end-of-life care between patient and health care team regarding treatment preferences, goals and location of care, through to formal, legally binding advance decisions to refuse treatment.
- Resources are now widely available to support ACP.[3–5]

End of life care

- Few patients with HF have been given the opportunity to discuss end of life care even if they have recognized death to be imminent.
- Sensitivity in communication requires skill and practice.
- Specific consideration needs to be given to changing the emphasis of treatment, starting or stopping treatment such as ICDs, resuscitation status, and 'do not attempt cardiopulmonary resuscitation' (DNACPR) orders (see 📖 Chapter 12).

Principles of effective communication

The term 'communication' encompasses a number of processes and skills:
- Imparting of information.
- Subtle balancing of benefits, burdens, and risks.
- Sensitivity and empathy.
- Honesty whilst maintaining hope and optimism.
- Telling the truth at a pace, and a level, tailored to the individual.
- Joint decision-making in complex situations of uncertainty.

Active listening, the ability to elicit patient concerns and to tailor the sharing of information and collaborative partnership in decision-making to individual patients, is a skill which is necessary and can be learned. How we communicate is as important as what we actually say.

Good communication results in:
- Promotion of trust.
- The opportunity for patients to make informed choices about treatment, their personal lives, and how and where they spend their time.

Poor communication can compound fear and anxiety and leave patients feeling more vulnerable and isolated.

Communication skills training

Acquiring the necessary skills in communication and negotiation requires training and support. Communication skills training offers the opportunity to learn a structured approach to communication and can lead to demonstrable improvement in attitudes, confidence, and skills.

Step-by-step models of sharing bad news are widely taught in medical schools and Foundation Programmes. Such models emphasize the need to pace discussions, in order that difficult information can be conveyed with the patient feeling that they have some control over the direction of the conversation and are not overwhelmed (see Table 4.1).

More advanced, intensive communication skills training can help professionals to hone their skills in managing the complexities of communicating with patients with advanced, progressive disease:
- How to tackle difficult subject matter, touching on personal and societal taboos.
- Discussion of complex information including risk and uncertainty.
- Negotiating the pace and timing at which information is shared. Patient preferences for degree of information and involvement in decision-making may fluctuate over time.
- Question assumptions made based on unreliable predictors such as age, culture, or educational background.

Communication is a process rather than a one-off event and involves:
- Recognition of when to respect a patient's right and need not to know whilst keeping the door open for open discussion in the future.
- Obtaining informed consent.
- Discussions with relatives.
- Eliciting and managing psychosocial concerns.
- Managing the emotions of patients and carers.

- Adapting an approach and prioritizing to meet the needs of frail palliative care patients.
- Making best interest decisions for patients lacking capacity.
- Managing one's own beliefs and fears about death and dying, and the impact on self of imparting bad news to others.

The support of a trusting ongoing patient-professional relationship is highly valued by patients and can be a powerful facilitator of effective communication. It can also aid the establishment of mutual expectations that is an important element of effective communication.

Table 4.1 Key points to consider when communicating important issues

Preparation	Clarify the purpose of the discussion
	Encourage the patient to bring a supportive relative or friend if wished
	Ensure sufficient time, comfort, and privacy
	Make sure you know the facts
	Make any necessary introductions
	Adopt a comfortable, listening posture—at the same level as the patient or relative
Communication	Ask open questions first
	Establish what the patient already knows
	Be open and honest; explain further if the patient wishes
	Elicit concerns, hopes, and fears; allow expression of emotion
	Maintain hope wherever possible. You can always offer the patient something: symptom control, psychological support, or practical help
	Avoid premature or unrealistic reassurance
	Clarify understanding
	Take the discussion at the patient's pace
	Involve the patient and carer in decision-making
	Summarize the discussion and plan
Follow-up	More than one consultation may well be necessary and preferable, depending on patient need

Table 4.1 (contd.)

	Different team members may be well placed to address differing aspects
	Provide a point of contact, e.g. nurse specialist
Documentation	Record the details in the medical notes
	Share information as necessary with others in the health care team, e.g. GP, nurse specialist, community matron

Adapted with permission from Kaye P (1996). *Breaking Bad News: A Ten Step Approach*. EPL, Northampton, p. 3.

Barriers to communication

The result of the many barriers to communication is that, by default, important discussions do not take place.

Potential barriers to communication may be present at all levels: patient, disease, professional, and organizational (see Table 4.2). One of the greatest barriers is the societal taboo on discussing death and dying, which applies equally to patients and professionals. In addition, many people with HF have significant comorbidities and the issues relating to the HF can be overlooked:

- The lack of a common language. For example, the term 'heart failure':
  - Is highly emotive, with the 'heart' often seen as central to life and sense of self.
  - Patients and clinicians can avoid using term perhaps because of the above.
  - Avoidance of the term may reflect, or lead to, insufficient information or explanation to properly understand their illness.
- Tacit acceptance by the patient of the professional agenda of 'balancing and monitoring' medication and physical symptoms can inhibit open discussion of their concerns, hopes, and priorities.
- The uncertainty due to the relapsing–remitting nature of, and increasing complexities of management options for, HF means that it can be difficult for clinicians to identify when sensitive discussions should be approached:
  - The possibility of death, especially sudden death, is often not discussed openly.
  - Not all patients are managed by cardiologists and many clinicians feel they have insufficient expertise to enter such discussions.
  - It is hard to know when treatment possibilities are appropriate or exhausted, or when to start discussing issues about advanced disease despite ongoing active measures.
- Health professionals have their own attitudes and emotions. They may feel:
  - Showing emotion or sympathy is not professional.
  - They may be blamed for the progression of the patient's illness.
  - Powerless in not being able to offer 'ready' cures.
  - Fear of unleashing an emotional reaction from the patient or their carers which they will find hard to manage.
  - Fear that distress itself may further harm the patient.
  - They should 'shield' the patient from bad news, to prevent distress or damaging hope.
  - Such emotions and thoughts can limit open communication between patient and professional.
- The 'mechanics' of the health care system can also act as a barrier to effective communication:
  - Lack of continuity of care.
  - Time constraints.
  - Patients may be reluctant to 'bother the busy doctor'.
  - Cardiologists may be understandably reluctant, or simply unable, to address the complexities of HF within a 10-minute appointment in a busy clinic.

Table 4.2 Barriers to communication

Patient- and disease-related factors	Difficulty in attending and participating in clinic appointments due to: symptoms such as breathlessness and fatigue; comorbidities such as dementia, poor eyesight and hearing; depression
	Lack of a 'common language'
	Tacit acceptance of professional agenda
	Cognitive impairment
	Relapsing/remitting nature of disease: difficulty with prognosis
	Societal taboo in discussing death and dying
Professional-related factors	No agreed single definition of the disease
	Perception that patients want prognostic certainty
	Don't want to upset patients
	See role solely as monitoring medical treatment
	Feeling of powerlessness
System-related factors	Poorly coordinated care especially between primary and secondary care
	Lack of planning and continuity of care
	Time constraints

Reprinted from Lawrie I and Kite S, Communication in Heart Failure, Table 7.1, pp. 93 in Johnson M and Lehman R (Eds), *Heart Failure and Palliative Care—A Team Approach*, Radcliffe Publishing Ltd, Oxford, 2006, with permission of Radcliffe Publishing Ltd.

Facilitators of effective communication in HF

General factors

The following factors have been found to facilitate communication with patients with advanced, progressive illness:[6]

- Patient experience of family/friends who have died.
- Trusting ongoing relationship with a doctor.
- Physician expertise in relevant specialty.
- Patient feeling cared for as a person.
- Doctor asks about end of life care skilfully.
- Patient has discussed end of life care with others previously.
- Patient experience of being very ill.
- Health system that expects doctors to have end of life discussions with patients.
- Advance care planning (see 📖 Chapter 8).

Addressing societal taboos

The Dying Matters Coalition is a national UK organization which aims to encourage people to talk about their wishes towards the end of their lives, including where they want to die and their funeral plans with friends, family and loved ones (http://www.dyingmatters.org/).

Engaging and empowering patients

Patients can be engaged and empowered in the management of their HF by approaches which place them firmly in control of their care:

- A question such as 'Who were you before you were ill?' can be a valuable tool for uncovering hopes, strengths, coping styles, and self-esteem.[7]
- Identifying and listing current problems can helps patients to recognize why they can feel so overwhelmed and act as a basis for prioritization of realistic goals.[6]

Communication of risk and uncertainty:

- Risk information can be presented in many ways including absolute risk, relative risk, percentages, odds and fractions.
- Patient preference and understanding varies.
- Try to avoid too many approaches in the same consultation.
- Question of 'risk of what?'. Doctors are likely to be focusing on risk of mortality and morbidity, whereas the patient's focus perspective may be on the likelihood of treatment restoring quality of life.

Coordination of communication

A coordinated service framework is necessary:

- Developed across an appropriate locality, e.g. citywide.
- Needs to describe how different professionals communicate with patients and each other and also who will take responsibility for the communication of specific aspects of care, including an assessment of psychosocial concerns.

- Ideally, identify a 'key worker' to take the lead in coordinating care across care settings, e.g. HF clinical nurse specialist or community matron.
- Mechanisms for home assessments or telephone consultations, where necessary, should be in place.

Communication in specific situations

Prognostication

The importance of this is clear, and communication is challenging:
- Prognostication is difficult, given the high degree of uncertainty in making individual predictions.
- Delay in addressing a deteriorating prognosis can deny the patient the opportunity to plan and make choices.
- Avoidance of discussion can cause distress for patients who suspect their poor prognosis.
- Timing: well and relatively symptom controlled patients may be unable or unwilling to consider the future. Acutely unwell patients may be more receptive but lack the energy, and the relevance of prognosis may diminish with health improvement.

Suggestions:
- Present the situation clearly and simply, outlining the stage in their illness the patient has reached, with some communication of risk.
- The use of simple statistics may be helpful for some, but not all, patients.
- Include options for treatment, care, and palliation of symptoms.
- Terms such as 'weeks to months', 'days to weeks', or 'hours to days' can convey useful timeframes—in general avoid greater specificity as this tends to be unreliable and are potentially damaging.

Withholding or withdrawing treatment

The following issues are important:
- A multidisciplinary assessment of the clinical benefit or otherwise of the intervention.
- An assessment of patient and caregiver wishes/understanding, including an assessment of the patient's mental capacity for any decisions they need to make.
- Adherence to mental capacity legislation[8] in the relevant jurisdiction for patients lacking capacity, and to relevant professional guidelines [e.g. GMC, British Medical Association (BMA)].
- Clarity of the aim of discussion:
  - To ascertain a patient's view on the advisability of an intervention which might potentially offer benefit?
  - To impart information about whether a particular intervention will or will not be offered?
- The discussion should be in the context of an overall consideration of stage of disease and plan of care.
- Be aware of the process required to manage conflict between clinical team and patient/caregiver:
  - Doctors are not obliged to offer physiologically futile interventions.
  - A second opinion may be needed, and can be supportive for all concerned.

CPR (see 📖 Chapter 12)

- CPR is an issue which patients may have considered and wish to talk about.
- It can act as a useful catalyst for discussion of future care.
- The clinician needs to be aware of up to date guidance from professional bodies and regulators, including mental capacity legislation.
- Discussion should take place with the patient (and family if the patient agrees) in the context of exploring an understanding of the patient's condition, their estimated prognosis, and the planned programme of care at this stage.
- Unrealistic expectations of the outcome in advanced disease are common:
  - Informed consent and refusal require understanding of the procedure, associated burdens, and chances of success.
  - Patients may define success differently from professionals.
- Make an individual decision:
  - Note that doctors are not obliged to offer medical treatments that have no chance of physiological success. Beware, the term 'futile' is pejorative to many, and may be interpreted as 'they don't think it's worth saving me'.
- The patient may be too unwell to participate. It is good practice to involve family and caregivers, making it clear that their views are taken into account, but that they do not carry responsibility for the decision:
  - reassure carers that they are not imposing a 'death sentence' by agreeing to a DNACPR order.

ICDs (see 📖 Chapter 12)

- ICDs are used in an attempt to prevent premature death due to ventricular arrhythmias.
- They may also prolong the dying process and make dying more distressing for the patient and those around them if not appropriately managed.
- Discussion regarding deactivation can be difficult as the patient's condition progresses and the end of life approaches.
- Patients and carers may have significant misconceptions, such as an association of ICDs with 'being kept alive', and of deactivation with immediate death.
- Ideally, the implications, advantages and disadvantages of both inserting and deactivating the device should be clearly discussed prior to ICD insertion.
- The patient's views will be informed by their experience of the results of previous ICD activation, if any.
- The patient may not appreciate that as disease progresses, the likelihood that an ICD prolongs survival lessens significantly.
- The timing of this discussion and subsequent deactivation is crucial, in general following a DNACPR order make decisions on an individual basis of overall benefit versus harm: there may be some 'grey' situations, e.g. where the potential for immediate defibrillation from an ICD in a geographically remote patient is chosen, although the likelihood of a successful outcome from delayed CPR is minimal.
- Informed patient choice is crucial.

Palliative and end of life care

- For timing of discussions see 📖 Chapters 3, 5, 7, and 8.
- Good communication in this context takes time, effort, and humility.
- The quality of communication can have a profound effect on the quality of remaining life and death for the patient, and for the bereavement experience of those close to them.
- In the last days of life The Liverpool Care Pathway for the Dying[9] (LCP) (or equivalent) covers key aspects of communication, along with physical, psychosocial, and spiritual aspects of care.

The role of family and carers

- Communication with family members or friends close to the patient is fundamental to palliative care.
- Such discussions must be with the permission of competent patients.
- Sometimes, family members insist on information being withheld from the patient, usually in an attempt to protect the patient from distress (collusion):
  - This is nearly always problematic and can distress the patient due to: non-verbal cues; loss of trust in their health care team and carers; prevention of informed choices; and suspicion of the truth with no outlet for clarification of their concerns and for exploration of fears.
  - Acknowledge the insights of family members, and tactfully explore the above.
- The role of the Lasting Power of Attorney is covered under advance care planning (see 📖 Chapter 8).
- Health professionals are expected to be conversant, and act in accordance with, mental health legislation and codes of practice in their jurisdiction.

References

1 General Medical Council (GMC) (2010) *Treatment and care towards the end of life: good practice in decision making.* GMC, London. http://www.gmc-uk.org/guidance/ethical_guidance/end_of_life_care.asp
2 Royal College of Physicians (2009) *Advance care planning. National guidelines.* RCP, London. http://bookshop.rcplondon.ac.uk/contents/pub267-e5ba7065-2385-49c9-a68e-f64527c15f2a.pdf
3 NHS End of Life Care (NEOLC) Programme: *Capacity, care planning and advance care planning in life limiting illness* (http://www.endoflifecareforadults.nhs.uk/assets/downloads/ACP_booklet_2011_Final_1.pdf).
4 Preferred priorities for care (http://www.endoflifecareforadults.nhs.uk/tools/core-tools/preferredprioritiesforcare).
5 Gold Standards Framework (http://www.goldstandardsframework.org.uk/).
6 Kite S (2010) Advance care planning. *Clin Med* **10**, 275–8.
7 Lawrie I, Kite S (2006) Connolly M (2005), Quoted in 'Communication in heart failure'. In *Heart failure and palliative care—a team approach* (ed. M Johnson, R Lehman), pp. 99–100. Radcliffe Publishing, Oxford.
8 HM Government (2005). Mental Capacity Act 2005. Code of Practice. http://www.dh.gov.uk/en/SocialCare/Deliveringsocialcare/MentalCapacity/MentalCapacityAct2005/index.htm
9 *Liverpool Care Pathway for the dying patient.* Marie Curie Palliative Care Institute, Liverpool. http://www.liv.ac.uk/mcpcil/liverpool-care-pathway/

Diagnosing end-stage heart disease

Introduction

The clinical course of HF has been transformed by therapies targeted at the underlying pathophysiology and the advent of VADs and cardiac transplantation. However, the ultimate outcome remains poor. End-stage disease may be prolonged and interspersed by periods of time when the patient seems improved. Symptom and caregiver burden is significant, and the timing of death can be difficult to predict.

An assessment of prognosis helps provide an important framework in which to weigh up the benefits and burdens of therapeutic interventions (see 📖 Chapter 3).

Comorbid disease may be the cause of death or contribute to it.

Recognition of the need for supportive and palliative care (see 📖 Chapter 6)

There are a number of markers that will help the clinician realize that their patient is in need of supportive care, particularly if one uses a modification of the 1990 WHO definition of palliative care substituting HF for cancer.

> The active total care of patients whose disease is not responsive to curative treatment. Control of pain, of other symptoms, and of psychological, social, and spiritual problems is paramount. The goal of palliative care is achievement of the best quality of life for patients and their families. Many aspects of palliative care are also applicable earlier in the course of the illness in conjunction with conventional care for the patient with HF.
>
> Modified from the WHO 1990 definition (http://www.who.int/cancer/palliative/definition/en/)

One helpful way to raise awareness in one's own practice is to ask the question 'Would you be surprised if this person were to die in the next 12 months?'. If the answer is 'no', the clinician should be considering if such a person has palliative care needs. Prognostication is a very inexact science. However, we know that clinicians overestimate prognosis more frequently than the converse. Therefore, if in doubt, the chances are the person does have a prognosis of less than 12 months. In the UK a general practice initiative, the GSF (http://www.goldstandardsframework.org.uk/), can help both identify patients and then improve their care.

The GSF

The aim of the GSF is to provide one gold standard for all end of life care. It is a programme for community palliative care, practice- or locality-based. It has a common sense framework that was initially developed for cancer care but is now recognized to be relevant to all with supportive and palliative care needs aiming to optimize the organization of and the quality of care. The key elements all involve communication and are patient-centred:

- Identify patients in need of palliative/supportive care.
- Assess their needs, symptoms, and preferences.
- Plan care around needs.

The goals of care are that the patient:

- Is symptom-free or at minimum has symptoms addressed.
- Identifies their preferred place of end of life care.
- Feels secure and supported by means of:
  - advance care planning (see 📖 Chapter 8),
  - addressing information needs,
  - knowledge that planned care will lead to fewer crisis admissions.

For carers and staff the gains are as follows.

- Carers are supported, enabled, and empowered to provide optimal care.
- Staff gain confidence through team working.

The seven Cs

The GSF identifies key tasks, known as the 'seven Cs'.

- Communication within primary care which includes:
  - a register of all patients with palliative care needs,
  - all such patients discussed at a multidisciplinary meeting,
  - improved discussion with patient to include advance care planning.
- Coordination of care with nomination of a co-coordinator.
- Control of symptoms, which should be:
  - assessed,
  - recorded,
  - acted on.
- Continuity, which includes out of hours (OOH) care:
  - systems put in place for OOH care.
- Continued learning by primary care.
- Carer support.
- Care of the dying phase:
  - diagnosing dying,
  - could use the integrated care pathway (see 📖 Chapter 13),
  - must use anticipatory prescribing.

Prognostic indicator

A prognostic indicator is being developed to aid the identification of adult patients with advanced disease in the last months or year of life, and those who are in need of supportive and palliative care. This encompasses the following:

General predictors of end-stage disease

- Multiple comorbidities (with no primary diagnosis).

- Weight loss greater than 10% over 6 months.
- General physical decline.
- Serum albumin < 25g/L.
- Reduced performance status/ KPS < 50%.
- Dependence in most activities of daily living (ADL).

Indicators specific to heart disease used by the GSF
At least two of the following:
- NYHA class III or IV.
- Hospital admissions due to HF.
- Thought by care team to be in the last year of life.
- Difficult/persistent physical or psychological symptoms despite optimal tolerated therapy.

Prognostic indices in HF (see also 📖 Chapter 3)

There are several scoring systems for prognostication in HF that include markers such as NYHA status, renal function, serum BNP levels, serum sodium levels, and cardiac cachexia.[1–4]

However, in practice, a patient who fulfils the GSF criteria above with progressive renal dysfunction, cardiac cachexia, escalating diuretic doses, and recurrent episodes of decompensation requiring hospital admission despite optimally tolerated therapy, or changes in biochemical markers, worsening performance status, and increasing symptoms is should have a full assessment for supportive and palliative care needs in recognition that they now have end-stage disease.

Barriers to diagnosing end-stage disease

- Fluctuating disease trajectory and daily variations in quality of life in the individual patient can make it difficult to predict which episode of deterioration signifies a change in disease status.
- Tendency for clinicians to continue to look for further treatment options even when these are futile.
- Clinician reluctance/lack of skills to discuss aims of treatment as disease progresses.
- Poor understanding of patient and caregiver regarding stage of illness.
- Repeated cycle of anxiety with deterioration followed by restoration with treatment makes it difficult for all to recognize when restoration is becoming less likely.

Importance of diagnosing end-stage disease

- Allows discussion with and support for patient and caregiver regarding preferred place of care and preferred place of death.[5]
- Even if there is sudden cardiac death at home, if the patient's wishes for a home death were known then inappropriate use of an emergency ambulance service may be prevented.
- Allows discussion about realistic hopes and aims of treatment, and treatment choice.
- Allows access to support (social services and financial), symptom control, and advance care planning and coordination of care (including OOH care).

Place of death

- Most patients, given the choice, would opt to die at home if their symptoms are controlled, their caregivers are supported, and their caregivers support their wish.
- Currently, most patients with cardiovascular disease die in hospital.[6]
- Even if a patient dies in hospital, either by choice or default, many deaths can be recognized and good care given by using tools such as the LCP or equivalent.[7]

Diagnosing dying—the terminal phase

The process of recognizing dying follows the principle of assessing a patient's current presentation within the context of their individual illness trajectory as discussed above (📖 Chapter 5, The GSF, pp. 62–3):

- Previous hospital admissions with decompensation.
- Not tolerating cardiac drugs—persistent hypotension.
- Persistent hyponatraemia despite optimizing diuretics.
- Worsening renal dysfunction.
- Increasing doses of diuretics with reducing or no response.
- Poor peripheral perfusion.
- Profound fatigue.
- Breathlessness at rest.
- Unable to take oral medication.
- Unable to manage more than sips of fluid.
- Reduced level of consciousness.
- Lack of response to intervention.

Clinicians will and should always assess to check that no reversible condition has been missed. However, it is also advisable, particularly with patients who are so ill, that where possible the patient is involved in the discussion about a management plan as they may have clear views on how much investigation and intervention they wish to undergo once they understand how unwell they are.

Some patients will have already realized that their prognosis is very poor and others will come to that understanding with gentle but open discussion (see 📖 Chapter 4). Such patients may well request comfort measures only, and if the discussion occurs in hospital, may request transfer home, if possible, so they can die there. Others may wish the clinician to continue with all possible treatments. This can cause difficulties when the patient requests a treatment which the clinician assesses as futile. GMC guidance is clear that a patient cannot demand a futile treatment, is equally clear that futile treatments do not have to be discussed with a patient, although good practice encourages discussion about the management plan in the context of what it is appropriate to offer (📖 Chapter 12, CPR, pp. 162–3 and Withdrawal of ICD support, pp. 164–6).

Where uncertainty remains, then tools such as the LCP can still be used as prompts of excellent care, but additional treatments that are clinically justified and regularly reviewed to assess response or not may still be given. If the patient subsequently dies, then they will have had good care during this time, and if the patient recovers they will have had good symptom control as they respond to treatment. Acknowledging the gravity of the illness, but also the uncertainty, to the patient and their caregivers is very appropriate management and does not prevent access to potentially helpful interventions.

Listening to the patient and family/carers

Patients and caregivers are likely to have concerns as they notice deterioration. HF patients have a tendency to attribute increasing symptoms and worsening performance status to the inevitable decline of aging and may not volunteer such concerns in the cardiology clinic. It is therefore vital that patients and caregivers are given the opportunity and confidence to raise worries with members of the primary or secondary care team. A regular open question at reviews such as 'how are things going?' may encourage disclosure, but often systematic assessment as described earlier (☐ Chapter 5, The GSF, pp. 62–3) is needed. The recent emphasis on keyworkers appears helpful, and in the UK the HF nurse specialists, who have often developed a strong therapeutic relationship over time, are well placed to fulfil this role.

The patient's and family's perspective

Patients come to the realization that they are dying in their own time and in their own way with a range of emotions and coping strategies accompanying this recognition. Worden's work on loss in the context of mourning explains the emotions patients experience as they are confronted with their own mortality and their passage through overlapping stages of coping from the time that they become aware of their prognosis until their actual death.[8] In order to be of help, we must first appreciate the enormous psychological impact dying has on the terminally ill patient and their family. Insight into the nature and range of coping mechanisms patients employ to manage the many powerful and sometimes conflicting emotions elicited by the prospect of death is paramount, as only by understanding this model of grief are we able to share the patient's unique journey and offer the most appropriate intervention. Patients express loss in different ways, rarely if ever progressing systematically through the stages of mourning but more frequently dipping in and out as they process newly acquired information. At such times it is helpful if their behaviour and emotions can be normalized within the framework of someone who is grieving not just for what they have lost, but also anticipatory grief for what they are about to lose.

The most commonly expressed emotions at this time are:
- Denial.
- Anger and despair that, if internalized, can manifest as depression.
- Difficulty in making decisions about future care pathways.
- Sadness that life is to end and goodbyes need to be said.
- Fear about the process of dying.
- Anxiety about those left behind and any business left unfinished.
- Ambivalence.
- Guilt and self-reproach—wondering if a change of lifestyle could have prevented progression of the disease.
- Isolation, often self-imposed, as a sense of 'aloneness' encompasses them.
- Helplessness and powerlessness—at not being able to change the inevitable course that their illness will take.

- Yearning for what was and what will never again be.
- Relief that the struggle will soon be over.
- Acceptance that death is inevitable.

The cardiologist's perspective

Recognizing and managing end-stage HF is as important as making the initial diagnosis of HF, establishing the aetiology and deciding on the most appropriate management plan for that patient. Often these components of HF care are done very well, but cardiologists are less good at recognizing and admitting when the focus of care should shift to being primarily related to symptom management. Missing the diagnosis of end-stage HF occurs due to a variety of reasons:

- Not all patients with HF are managed by a cardiologist.
- Many patients have HF in addition to other comorbidities and it may not be recognized that the HF has caused the clinical decline.
- Unpredictable illness trajectory with multiple episodes of decline and recovery make recognizing end-stage HF difficult and off-putting as doctors don't want to feel 'they got it wrong' and patients will often feel they recovered once so could do so again.
- Therapeutic strategies for HF have become more varied and complex, so that it is hard to feel sure that all options have been exhausted unless one specializes in this area.
- Cardiologists are used to being able to 'do things that make patients better' and therefore there is the tendency to keep trying something else even when the inevitable seem obvious.
- Tendency to focus on the 'here and now' and not on the longer term.
- Patients with HF are often referred from other teams as a complication from another severe/significant illness and as such there is often an expectation from the referring team, patient, and/or relatives that 'something can be done'. Its therefore very difficult to say 'no' to the patient and family immediately, which can then start a spiral of investigations and interventions which may not be ultimately appropriate.
- Many cardiologists are not adequately trained to share bad news with patients and are therefore hesitant about having these conversations.
- Patients with HF are often admitted to hospital OOH when their usual care team is not available, and as such it is understandably difficult to be the on-call cardiologist and have 'end of life' discussions with a patient unknown to that doctor. These conversations are time-consuming and OOH there is often not the capacity for these types of conversations to occur with patients and their families.

References

1 Koelling TM, Joseph S, Aaronson KD (2004) Heart failure survival score continues to predict clinical outcomes in patients with heart failure receiving beta-blockers. *J Heart Lung Transplant* **23**, 1414–22.

2 Lee DS, Austin PC, Rouleau JL, Liu PP, Naimark D, Tu JV (2003) Predicting mortality among patients hospitalized for heart failure: derivation and validation of a clinical model. *J Am Med Assoc* **290**, 2581–7.

3 Levy WC, Mozaffarian D, Linker DT et al. (2006) The Seattle Heart Failure Model: prediction of survival in heart failure. *Circulation* **113**, 1424–33.

4 Senni M, Santilli G, Parrella P et al. (2006) A novel prognostic index to determine the impact of cardiac conditions and co-morbidities on one-year outcome in patients with heart failure. *Am J Cardiol* **98**, 1076–82.

5 Johnson M, Parsons S, Raw J, Williams A, Daley A (2009) Achieving preferred place of death – is it possible for patients with chronic heart failure? *Br J Cardiol* **16**, 194–6.

6 Office for National Statistics (ONS) (2009) *Mortality statistics: general.* DH1 No 36 2003. (http://www.statistics.gov.uk/downloads/theme_health/Dh1_36_2003/DH1_2003.pdf)

7 *Liverpool Care Pathway for the dying patient.* Marie Curie Palliative Care Institute, Liverpool. (http://www.liv.ac.uk/mcpcil/liverpool-care-pathway/)

8 Worden JW (1991). *Grief counseling and grief therapy.* Springer, New York.

Chapter 6

Integrating supportive and palliative care

Introduction

- People with HF need access to supportive and palliative care.
  However, barriers remain and the prolonged burden for sufferers and
  their carers are still unalleviated for many.
- Recognition of the transition to end-stage disease seems to be a key
  problem (see 📖 Chapters 1, 3, and 5).

Therefore, a problem-centred approach, according to need or capacity
to benefit rather than one dependent upon diagnosis or clear prognosis,
appears to be useful, allowing provision of supportive and palliative
care alongside and integrated with appropriate interventions for the HF
itself.[1,2]

In addition, specialist palliative care services should then discharge
HF patients from their services if the issues are resolved, thus fostering
confidence that patients can 'dip in and out of' appropriate care and start
to move away from traditional views of referral being necessarily a 'one-
way ticket'.

Such an integrated approach maintains the often strong relationship
between patient and clinicians in both primary and secondary care and may
prevent the reluctance that can accompany a referral that is associated
with a handing over of care.

The need for supportive and palliative care[3]

Patients with HF are disadvantaged compared with patients with cancer with regard to the following:

- They have a similar symptom burden but are less likely to have access to supportive and palliative care services, especially specialist palliative care services.
- They have less understanding of their illness.
- They are less likely to have their informational, psychosocial, emotional and spiritual needs addressed.
- They are less likely to be involved in advance care planning for their own illness and place of care/death.

Triggers for supportive and palliative care

Disease trajectory triggers (see also 📖 Chapter 3)

Population studies describe the trajectory of chronic HF as gradual decline, punctuated by episodes of acute deterioration, which may result in recovery, or death, which is still seen as sudden.

Three broad key stages have been suggested: chronic disease management, supportive and palliative care, and the dying phase.[4]

Change in trajectory stage

- A 'sentinel' event such as hospital admission could be a trigger to change from chronic disease management to supportive and palliative care.[4]
- NYHA class and KPS have been suggested as indications of stage, e.g. NYHA I–II, KPS 80–100% as chronic disease management, NYHA III–IV, KPS 50–70% as supportive and palliative care and NYHA IV or KPS <50% as the dying phase.[4]
- Individuals may, of course, follow a totally chaotic trajectory, and any trigger should be flexible enough to allow access to palliative care services, but also discharge from palliative services. As illustrated by the case history, HF patients can respond to supportive and palliative care measures so well that their performance status and NYHA class improve.
- Failure to recognize that leads back into the 'prognostic paralysis' of the clinician feeling they have to be *certain* that the patient has entered a particular stage before they may be referred to palliative care services.

Co-ordination of care

The 'revolving door' admission

Although the HF nurse specialist (HFNS) has had a significant impact on such admissions, nevertheless this situation is an example of a trigger for assessing the need for supportive and palliative care. If this is not done, the patient may be admitted under a different receiving physician and the overall plan of care lost.

- There is a need for exemplary communication between primary and secondary care, and between clinician, patient, and caregiver.
- Patients appreciate a clear plan of care on discharge from hospital communicated to them and their primary care team.
- The emphasis during the hospital admission tends to be on restoring fluid balance rather than taking an overall view of the patient's needs.
- Therefore the in-hospital attending team must take the time to gain an in-context impression of the patient's pre-decompensation performance status lest inappropriate and futile interventions be attempted.

Assessing areas of concern

People with HF experience supportive and palliative care needs in all domains of their lives, therefore any assessment should be holistic.

Although this is routine care in oncology and can be done using simple assessment tools which can be incorporated into standard clinic time,[5] there is still some way to go in cardiac clinics or primary care. The assessment should include the patient's caregiver where present.

Areas to assess[5]

- Unresolved physical symptoms (e.g. breathlessness, fatigue, sleeping, pain, nausea).
- Problems with ADL.
- Psychological, emotional, or spiritual concerns.
- Financial or legal concerns.
- Are there health beliefs, social or cultural aspects, or family aspects that contribute to the complexity of care?
- Family function and caregiver wellbeing.
- Need for referral for further assessment or to supportive or palliative care agency.

Repeated assessment

- Assessment needs to be repeated and conversations revisited.
- This allows for a patient's conditions to improve as well as deteriorate and for a patient to change their mind about treatment or place of care.
- This ensures that management options to remain appropriate for the patient's clinical condition and likely prognosis (both for the patient who improves more than expected and the one who deteriorates more than expected).

Case history

Presentation

Mr D was 38 years old when he was referred to the palliative care consultant. He had chronic degenerative back pain following a road traffic accident in his late teens. He has smoked heavily since he was 9 years old, had his first myocardial infarction at 27, and a coronary artery bypass graft at 30. He developed chronic HF at 32 and was stable on optimal medical management until he was 35. However, he now has NYHA III HF, and is only tolerating ramipril 2.5mg at night (nocte) because of hypotension. When seen in the palliative care clinic, he had the following issues:

- Physical:
  - Back pain felt in his lower back, worse on standing for more than a few minutes. This was the reason for him getting a wheelchair but now he needs it because he is so breathless.
  - He is breathless on minimal exertion. At night he cannot lie flat, waking after getting to sleep having slipped down the pillows after about 30 minutes. This wakes his wife so both are very tired.
  - Fatigued and drowsy in the day.
- Financial. He is self-employed. At the moment he is unable to work, but has no sickness insurance. He is heavily in debt and can't sleep because of all this worry.

- Family. He has a 5-year-old son and an 8-year-old daughter. He met his son from nursery one day and collapsed in front of him; since then his son has been frightened to be alone in the house with him, and won't even sit on his knee. The older child has been in a lot of trouble at school. His wife says she's at the end of 'her rope' and thinking of leaving but it would be like 'leaving a puppy that's been run over'.
- Psychological. He freely admits he is depressed. He has no concentration. He has lost his role in the family. As he can't work, this is feeding his loss of sense of self. He has also lost his libido and is worried he is losing his wife and thence his children.
- Spiritual: 'I'm too young to be like this', 'what's it all been for anyway?', 'it's all my fault'.

Management
- 8 weeks day hospice to allow regular assessment and review with the multiprofessional team and some time out for his wife.
- Child and adolescent counsellor for the children.
- Occupational therapy assessment (electric wheelchair for outside only to get him out of the house, other practical aids for daily living in the house including a profiling bed to stop him slipping down the pillows at night).
- Pain management—opioids, physiotherapy, tricyclic antidepressant, supportive care.
- Breathlessness management—opioids, physiotherapy (exercise!) and fan, diuretic optimization.
- Psychological management—supportive care, tricyclic antidepressant.
- Spiritual management—access to hospice chaplaincy, but chose to talk with hospice staff in general.
- Financial review with benefits advice and debt management.
- Creative writing programme—bedtime story writing for children.
- Review of local adult learning opportunities.

Outcome
- Needed second 8-week day hospice attachment.
- Had concurrent referral for transplant consideration—turned down.
- Back pain controlled.
- Mobility improved with physiotherapy, pain control, and breathlessness control.
- With improved mobility, cardiorespiratory reserve improved.
- As mobility improved, blood pressure improved, his ACE inhibitor could be up-titrated to the target dose.
- The children did well with the counselling, and the younger one was delighted to feature in the bedtime story that was written.
- His mood improved and so has his relationship with his wife and family.
- He attempted to go to computer classes, but this was not successful; however, he remains more optimistic, and has become involved in a local charity in order to feel more useful.

- His finances remain rather precarious but he is on a debt management programme and he feels more in control.
- He is now NYHA II and has been discharged from the specialist palliative care services.

Key people to integrate supportive and palliative care

The HFNS

- HFNSs are well placed to act as key workers for patients, making detailed holistic patient assessments and liaising across services to ensure the many needs are met.
- A national survey conducted by the National Council for Palliative Care in 2005 and repeated in 2010 showed that HFNSs felt they had a vital role to play in providing general palliative care for their HF patients and in liaising with the specialist palliative care services for those with persistent and complex symptoms.[6]
- HFNSs value easy access to specialist palliative care health professionals, and formalized pathways of care between cardiology and palliative care. Where the nurses worked in services with formal referral criteria, these nurses referred more patients to the palliative care services.
- Most HFNS services now have access to specialist palliative care services, although there still appears to be some way to go before the inequity of access compared with cancer patients is truly addressed.

GPs

GPs are also key providers of general supportive and palliative care services for people with HF throughout their illness. They:
- Are well placed to perform holistic assessment and ongoing care.
- Recognize the need for coordinated, advanced planning with good continuity of care but appreciate confirmation and clear communication from colleagues in secondary care when a patient has reached end-stage disease.
- Need clarity regarding which clinician holds overall responsibility for care.

Suggested transition points to consider reassessment of supportive and palliative care needs

- At diagnosis: information about the diagnosis and prognosis needs to be tailored to the individual.
- As new treatments are considered: for example, at the time an ICD is inserted, the clinician should assess whether discuss deactivation of the device is possible.
- As chronic HF becomes end stage—transition from NYHA III to NYHA IV. The aims of care should be discussed as the patient allows. The major focus will be on palliation but continued optimization of tolerated chronic HF therapies will remain important within this for symptom control.
- As cardiac medication becomes more difficult to tolerate, e.g. the dose of ACE inhibitor has to be reduced because of hypotension. Full assessment of symptom burden, understanding of stage of disease, and preferences for place of care should be sensitively explored.
- After every hospital admission for decompensated chronic HF. This should trigger a review of where the patient is on the disease trajectory preferably performed by the GP informed by the secondary care physician and HFNS.
- When it appears that the patient is at the end of life, when a further deterioration is failing to respond to remedial treatment, a full reassessment of needs and understanding will enable appropriate care of the dying.

What's needed?

Integrating cardiology and supportive and palliative care services is not necessarily straightforward, although some areas of the UK now have established services. Where services have succeeded, the following areas have been addressed:

- Mutual education and support, e.g. palliative care multidisciplinary team meetings, education meetings, joint clinics, ward visits, consultations.
- Local protocols in place, e.g. referral criteria and pathways, reprogramming of ICDs, administration of subcutaneous furosemide.
- Advanced communication skills in place for the cardiology team, e.g. the British Heart Foundation has funded places for UK cardiology staff to attend courses.
- Change in mindset towards a holistic assessment of the patient rather than purely evidence based titration of cardiac medications.

Summary

- Integration of palliative care, cardiology, and primary care services is required.
- Basic skills of supportive and palliative care needs assessment, with excellent communication skills, are vital for cardiology and primary care teams.
- An awareness of triggers that may indicate transition to end-stage disease, but are flexible enough to allow for patient recovery, will lead to a problem-based approach providing appropriate and timely palliative care whilst leaving the door open for relevant cardiac interventions.
- Referrals to specialist palliative care should be for persistent or complex issues, with the option of discharge from the service if resolution occurs.
- Integration should be *problem* based rather than *prognosis* based.

References

1 Goodlin SJ, Hauptman PJ, Arnold R et al. (2004) Consensus statement: palliative and supportive care in advanced heart failure. *J Card Failure* **10**, 200–9.

2 Jaarsma T, Beattie JM, Ryder M et al. (2009) Palliative care in heart failure: a position statement from the palliative care workshop of the Heart Failure Association of the European Society of Cardiology. *Eur J Heart Failure* **11**, 433–43.

3 Murray SA, Boyd K, Kendall M, Worth A, Benton TF, Clausen H (2002) Dying of lung cancer or cardiac failure: prospective qualitative interview study of patients and their carers in the community. *BMJ* **325**, 929.

4 Boyd KJ, Worth A, Kendall M et al. (2009) Making sure services deliver for people with advanced heart failure: a longitudinal qualitative study of patients, family carers, and health professionals. *Palliat Med* **23**, 767–76.

5 Waller A, Girgis A, Lecathelinais C et al. (2010) Validity, reliability and clinical feasibility of a needs assessment tool for people with progressive cancer. *Psychooncology* **19**, 726–33.

6 Johnson MJ, MacCallum A, Butler J et al. (2011) Heart failure specialist nurses' use of palliative care services: a comparison of surveys across England in 2005 and 2010. *Eur J Cardiovasc Nurs* doi:10.1016/j.ejcnurse.2011.03.004

Chapter 7

Optimizing management in end-stage HF

Introduction

Tailored therapy, self-management programmes, and keyworker support from nurse specialists have transformed the care of patients with HF over the past 10–15 years. Guidelines for pharmacological and device management have been developed and service frameworks such as the National Service Framework for Coronary Heart Disease[1] have improved services and outlook for patients.

In end-stage disease, HF management is challenging as individuals may not be able to tolerate standard recommended medications such as ACE inhibitors or ARBs, beta-blockers, aldosterone antagonists (AAs), and H-ISDN. Thus, although the guidelines are helpful, they need to be applied to each patient and reviewed regularly. In addition, as patients deteriorate they may find their tablet burden excessive, and rationalizing treatment with symptom relief as the focus rather than long-term reduction of risk is required.

Polypharmacy

- Regularly review all medications and stop any that are unnecessary for symptom control. (Remember that ACE inhibitors, ARBs, beta-blockers and AAs are beneficial for symptom control as well as survival, and should therefore be continued as tolerated.)
- Review the side-effect:benefit ratio for each patient.
- Consider the patient's view on difficulty in taking prescribed medications.
- Patients with HF often have several comorbidities, treatment for which adds to the medication burden; the same consideration should be given for non-cardiac medications.

Diuretics

Use: management of fluid balance and symptom management only. No prognostic benefit.

Mode of administration: oral, subcutaneous (SC), IV.[*]

Dose: as required to manage fluid overload. (Resistant fluid overload management should be discussed with the local cardiologist.)

- Patients with renal dysfunction often require higher doses.
- Patients may require a parenteral loop diuretic when they have become fluid overloaded such that oral absorption is impaired.

Diuretic increase

- As needed to modify symptoms of breathlessness associated with fluid overload and peripheral oedema.
- Many patients will be familiar with a self-management programme of increasing their own oral loop diuretic if their weight has increased and will have been instructed when to contact the HF nurse for further advice.

Alternative diuretic strategies for worsening or resistant symptoms

- Addition of thiazide diuretic, e.g. bendroflumethiazide or metolazone, to a loop diuretic.
- High-dose oral diuretic with tds dosing rather than single-dose increases.
- Switch loop diuretics, e.g. furosemide to bumetanide—this may allow increased gastrointestinal absorption, especially in the presence of gut oedema.

Diuretic reduction

- Clinical dehydration (postural drop in blood pressure with accompanying symptoms of fatigue and faintness on standing; thirst, reduced skin turgor, reduced jugular venous pressure).
- Uraemia.
- Patients ask for this if distressed by frequency of micturition.
- Some patients require a 'diuretic holiday'. Diuretic holidays are used primarily for patients who require diuretics to control fluid overload but who become clinically and biochemically dry The patient is given a period of time (often 24–72hr) diuretic free with assessment of fluid balance and biochemistry allowing for adjustments of the diuretics as needed.

---

[*] A decision needs to be made by the main care team regarding the ceiling of appropriate medical therapy as this will influence the route of administration which might in turn affect the option of locations as to where the care can take place.

Disease-modifying medications

Mode of administration: oral.
Dose: maximally tolerated aiming for target dose specific to each drug.

Disease-modifying medications are prescribed in all patients with HF unless there is a valid contraindication as the following benefits have been clearly demonstrated:
• Survival.
• Reduction in hospital admission for HF.
• Improvement in symptoms and quality of life.

Most patients tolerate these medications well.
• Problems such as renal dysfunction or hypotension are usually only seen with initiation of the drug, or with very end stage disease. Problems can arise when the patient is acutely unwell with HF or sepsis. With the latter any HF medications stopped during this phase should be restarted where possible and a further trial of tolerance given.
• Even if a patient has reached a 'palliative phase', disease-modifying medications should continue at the highest dose that does not cause persistent symptomatic hypotension or other side-effects such as renal impairment or bradycardia, as many improve symptoms.
• Continual assessment and review is important as the patient may be variable in their ability to tolerate these drugs, and adjustments in medications are likely to be needed.
• In people with precarious blood pressure, the drugs may need to be temporarily stopped or the dose reduced to allow sufficient diuretic dose to be given to address fluid overload. It is important to go back to the maximum tolerated dose once the acute episode is resolved.

Asymptomatic hypotension
• In the non-acute phase no adjustments need to be made if the patient feels well.
• Ensure the patient is not dehydrated.

Symptomatic hypotension
• Try nocturnal dosing.
• Ensure the patient is not dehydrated.
• If no improvement with nocturnal dosing reduce other hypotensive agents (specifics will depend on the patient and their comorbidities):
  • Reduce nitrate if angina stable.
  • If angina is a predominant feature reduce ACE inhibitors and/or ARBs in preference to a beta blocker or nitrate.
  • If atrial or ventricular arrhythmias a feature then reduce ACE inhibitors and or ARBs in preference to a beta blocker.
• H-ISDN is contraindicated in symptomatic hypotension.

Renal failure

Progressive renal impairment is common in advanced HF and the cause is usually multifactorial with medications, relative hypotension, and poor perfusion contributing to the cardiorenal disease process. In advanced HF deteriorating renal function is a poor prognostic indicator especially if resistant to reduction in medications such as ACE inhibitors, ARBs, AAs and diuretics or if the renal dysfunction is poor enough to necessitate that these medications are not restarted.

Renal impairment: general measures

Ensure adequate hydration:
- Consider a 'diuretic holiday' if appropriate.
- Review and stop any non-cardiac nephrotoxic agents, e.g. non-steroidal anti-inflammatory drugs (NSAIDS).
- Consider possible side-effects of medications reliant on renal metabolism, e.g. bisoprolol, digoxin, and low molecular weight heparin (LMWH) and reduce dose or stop accordingly.

Renal impairment without hyperkalaemia (regular monitoring should be in place)[2]

- Creatinine up to 50% baseline or < 266µmol/L—continue ACE inhibitor, ARB, AA.
- Creatinine > 266µmol/L but < 310µmol/L—half dose ACE inhibitor, ARB, and/or AA.
- Creatinine > 310µmol/L—stop ACE inhibitor, ARB, and/or AA.

Renal impairment with hyperkalaemia

- K^+ > 5.5mmol/L but < 6mmol/L:
  - reduce dose of ACE inhibitor, ARB, or AA
  - stop any potassium supplements.
- $K^+ \geq$ 6mmol/L:
  - stop ACE inhibitor, ARB, AA.
  - stop any potassium supplements.
- H-ISDN is contraindicated in renal failure.

Other factors

Symptomatic bradycardia
- Consider 12-lead ECG to exclude heart block or symptomatic pauses (if appropriate). If heart block or symptomatic pauses present then reduce/stop rate-limiting medication in first instance. If persists despite stopping rate-limiting medication then consider permanent pacemaker implantation.
- If symptomatic bradycardia only (no heart block or pauses):
  - reduce digoxin in preference to beta-blocker if prescribed both,
  - otherwise reduce beta-blocker.

Worsening HF
- Increase diuretic therapy and consider a reduction in beta-blocker dose.
- If tolerated, try and keep at least a small dose of ACE inhibitor as this may increase the effectiveness of the diuretic.

Device therapy and arrhythmia management

Device therapy needs to be continuously reviewed:

- For patients who remain symptomatic despite CRT it is important to assess if CRT optimization is appropriate and if it has been attempted. This is a procedure using echocardiography in which the CRT programming can be manipulated to work more effectively. Despite this some patients will remain symptomatic.

- For those with a defibrillator either in isolation (ICD) or in combination with CRT (CRTD) the appropriateness of the defibrillator remaining active and device programming needs to be reviewed regularly. A defibrillator monitors the heart rhythm and functions to treat ventricular arrhythmias with either anti-tachycardia pacing or shock therapy. A defibrillator can also function as a pacemaker if needed for bradycardia pacing. Where the defibrillator remains active the aim is to minimize the VT burden and the subsequent appropriate shocks.

- Medications such as amiodarone, beta blockers, and occasionally mexiletine are continued in patients who have regular episodes of VT who are still able to take oral medication. This is to prevent symptomatic distressing arrhythmias or shocks in people with ICDs. Mexiletine is a class IB anti-arrhythmic and is only prescribed by cardiologists to minimize the VT burden in the context of severe left-ventricular systolic dysfunction where other medications have been tried unsuccessfully.

- For some patients anti-tachycardia pacing can avoid or minimize shock therapy, therefore review of device programming should occur after any discharge.

- For patients who have discharges from their device it is important to establish that the shocks were appropriate. Patients at times can receive inappropriate shocks for other arrhythmias such as atrial fibrillation (AF) where the ventricular rate is fast enough to be detected within the VT zone of the defibrillator. This can usually be avoided with a combination of rate-limiting medications to control the rate of the arrhythmia and reprogramming of the device detection zones for VT.

Optimizing HF management appropriately for end of life care

Patients who are deteriorating clinically towards 'end of life care' (i.e. moving from Boyd's Phase 2 to 3 or who are already in Phase 3;[3] see 📖 Chapter 3, Escaping 'prognostic paralysis', pp. 38–9), this and discussions about plans for care at this stage will signal another review of their HF management:

- Where possible oral medications should be kept to a minimum and used only to modify symptoms. As such diuretic therapy (IV, oral, or SC) is often critical particularly for breathlessness associated with pulmonary oedema.
- Morphine (IV, oral, or SC) can be used very successfully as an adjunct to diuretic therapy for the relief of breathlessness and sublingual (SL) lorazepam for the anxiety associated with dyspnoea (see 📖 Chapters 9, 10, and 13).
- Disease-modifying medications should be reviewed on a regular basis.
    - For those patients in Phase 2, these medications should be continued where possible but stopped or reduced where the side-effects such as symptomatic hypotension or significant renal dysfunction outweigh the potential benefits.
    - For those patients in Phase 3 disease-modifying medications should be stopped at this point as they afford very little benefit.
- Beta blockers and digoxin should also be stopped in Phase 3 unless they are prescribed for the control of arrhythmias which if present would increase the symptom burden for the patient and the oral route is still possible.
- Amiodarone (oral or IV) is often prescribed for control of ventricular arrhythmias such as VT. Amiodarone (oral or IV) should be continued for as long as possible where patients have a high VT burden.
    - In Phase 3 where a patient is no longer able to swallow oral medications and the intravenous route is inappropriate then the amiodarone should be stopped.
    - Amiodarone has a long half life (90 days) and as such for patients in Phase 3 there should allow for adequate control of ventricular arrhythmias.
- Most patients in Phase 3 will not survive any ventricular arrhythmia and will become unconscious very quickly; however, anticipatory prescribing should include midazolam and morphine to manage any ventricular arrhythmias where the patient remains conscious.

The need for continuing anticoagulation is dependent on the requirement for warfarin, the phase of the patient's illness and other comorbidities adding to the falls risk and risk of bleeding from the gastrointestinal tract. For all patients there is an ongoing requirement to assess the risk:benefit ratio of warfarin.

- For patients in Phase 2 then continuation of warfarin is largely dependent on the initial need for warfarin.
- Patients prescribed warfarin for AF alone can stop warfarin more easily than those prescribed warfarin due to a prosthetic valve.

- For patients in Phase 2 prescribed warfarin for AF then the warfarin should be stopped at a time when the risk outweighs the benefit and replaced with aspirin.
- Patients in Phase 2 prescribed warfarin due to the presence of a prosthetic valve or pulmonary embolus do require anticoagulation, and as such if the risk of warfarin outweighs the benefit then the warfarin should be replaced with subcutaneous LMWH which can also be given in the community.
- Neither warfarin nor LMWH is required for patients in Phase 3 who are dying.

Breathlessness is usually managed with a combination of diuretic and opioids and titrated in order to control symptoms.
- In Phase 3 where breathlessness remains an issue then diuretics can be given subcutaneously via a syringe driver and titrated as required.
- The empirical dose of SC furosemide is equivalent to the previously prescribed oral or IV dose.
- Furosemide will not prolong life at this stage and is used purely as a method of palliating symptoms of breathlessness or distressing peripheral oedema.
- Where anxiety is a prominent feature of breathlessness and is not controlled with opioids then benzodiazepines can be used in addition.

Complex device therapy and end of life care

The devices of all patients with HF should be continually reviewed and the concept of defibrillator deactivation considered. The specific considerations of complex device therapy and end of life care are discussed in 📖 Chapter 12.

Intra-aortic balloon pumps (IABPs)

IABPs are used to augment diastolic BP resulting in improved coronary and cerebral perfusion without an increase in myocardial oxygen demand which tends to occur with inotropes. IABPs are often used in the following situations:
- Cardiogenic shock.
- Acute ventricular septal or valve rupture following MI.
- Bridge to cardiac transplantation.

In circumstances where the clinical situation is irrecoverable with no exit strategy (e.g. LVAD or cardiac transplant) and as such the IABP is no longer felt to be in the best interests of the patient, the IABP is weaned and then removed. The majority of patients will be IABP dependent and will die quickly after removal. This therefore needs to be discussed with the patient and family and appropriate anticipatory prescribing put in place.

Further reading

Arrhythmia Alliance Implantable cardioverter defibrillators (ICDs) in dying patients (http://www.hruk.org.uk/Docs/ICD%20Deactivation%20Leaflet-Arrhythmia%20Alliance.pdf).

References

1 National Service Framework for Cardiac Disease (2000) *Coronary heart disease.* Chapter 6 Heart failure. Available at: http://www.dh.gov.uk/prod_consum_dh/groups/dh_digitalassets/@ dh/@en/documents/digitalasset/dh_4057523.pdf.

2 Boyd KJ, Worth A, Kendall M et al. (2009) Making sure services deliver for people with advanced heart failure: a longitudinal qualitative study of patients, family carers, and health professionals. *Palliat Med* **23**, 767–76.

3 Dickstein K, Cohen-Solal A, Filippatos G et al. (2008) ESC guidelines for the diagnosis and treatment of acute and chronic heart failure 2008: the Task Force for the Diagnosis and Treatment of Acute and Chronic Heart Failure 2008 of the European Society of Cardiology. Developed in collaboration with the Heart Failure Association of the ESC (HFA) and endorsed by the European Society of Intensive Care Medicine (ESICM). *Eur Heart J* **29**, 2388–442.

Advance care planning (ACP)

Introduction

ACP is a voluntary process whereby patients can express their preferences and goals for future care *in advance of* the event that they lose capacity. It is a valuable way for enhancing communication within a group of patients for whom competence for decision-making may decline with increasing frailty and disease progression. Exploring preferences for future care, in the context of individual beliefs and values, and conveying these to carers and professionals, as well as family and friends, is an important component of palliative care, and such conversations usually take place during everyday clinical care. Knowledge of patients' values and beliefs can also guide best-interest decisions when unforeseen events occur.

ACP—summary issues

- A *process* of discussion about future care between an individual, their care providers, and often those close to them.
- A framework to inform health professionals' decision-making should the patient lose capacity.
- Spans the documentation of conversations that happen as apart of good end of life care between the patient and health care team regarding treatment preferences, goals, and location of care, through to formal, legally binding advance decisions.
- Excellent guidelines (RCP[1]), resources (NEOLC programme[2]), and tools (e.g. preferred priorities for care) are available.
- Opportunity to record advance decisions to refuse treatment in specific circumstances.
- Resuscitation status.
- Patient's preferred place of care and place of death.

ACP documents should be:
- Accessible at the point of care.
- Reviewed on a regular basis by the medical care team and kept up to date to reflect any changes as the clinical situation evolves.
- Referred to by health care professionals or family carers in the event that the patient loses the capacity to decide once their illness progresses.
- With permission, documented, regularly reviewed, and communicated with key people involved in care as an ACP record

Outcomes of ACP

Mental capacity legislation[3] stipulates that there are three types of documented outcomes in ACP:
- Advance statements.
- Advance decisions to refuse treatment (ADRT).
- Appointment of lasting power of attorney (LPA)/welfare power of attorney (WPA).[*]

---

[*] Terminology may vary between jurisdictions.

In addition the patient may wish to name a person whom they wish to be consulted in the event that they lose capacity

Advance statements (Box 8.1)

- Written statements either by the patient or written down for them with their agreement about their feelings and wishes whilst they have capacity regarding issues of their care that they *would wish* to be considered in the future should they lose capacity due to illness.
- Advance statements include:
  - Type of medical treatment they would want or not want.
  - Preferred place of care and preferred place of death.
  - How they wish to be cared for.
  - They are not the same as ADRTs.
  - They are not legally binding, but carers under the Mental Capacity Act[3] are required to take them into account when considering an individual's best interests.

Box 8.1 Advance statement summary

- Advance statement of preferences and wishes.
- Formalizes what patients and families *do* wish to happen.
- Helps clinicians plan care.
- Not legally binding.
- Related to other matters:
  - Mental Capacity Act
  - LPA.

ADRTs (Box 8.2)

- Previously known as living wills or advance directives.
- States what a patient does *not* want to happen to them and must relate to a specific treatment and a specific circumstance.
- Applicable when the patient loses capacity to consent to or refuse treatment.
- A competent (at the time of writing) adult's ADRT (e.g. CPR) is legally binding if it meets the conditions stipulated in the Mental Capacity Act 2005 (England & Wales).[3]
- An ADRT for life-sustaining treatment must be in writing, signed, and witnessed, and state that it applies *even if life is at risk*.
- Restrictions apply, e.g. basic nursing care cannot be refused, and inappropriate, clinically futile treatments, or illegal actions (such as physician-assisted suicide) cannot be demanded.
- A useful tool to support, but does not replace, discussion with patients and their carers to develop an overall picture of their wishes and preferences.
- Does not mean that treatment is being stopped now. Only comes into force in the future if the person concerned lacks capacity and the clinical situation is as described in the advance decision.
- Responsibility for keeping and presenting the advance decision or ACP lies with the patient.

- Rarely used with the exception of DNACPR orders because:
  - few people complete them
  - sufficient evidence of validity may not be available at the time of need (e.g. in Accident and Emergency (A&E)).

To be valid the doctor needs to be sure that:
- These were the wishes of this particular patient.
- That they were competent to make this particular decision at the time of writing the directive.
- That the directive refers specifically to the decision in question.
- That there is no evidence of the patient having changed their mind in the interim or having been subject to coercion.

Specific situations can rarely be predicted in sufficient detail to cover the reality at hand.

Box 8.2 ADRT summary

- Formalizes what patients do *not* want to happen.
- Legally binding (care with wording/situation etc.).
- Related to other matters:
  - Mental Capacity Act[3]
  - LPA

Power of attorney (POA)

An individual with capacity can appoint a POA to make decisions for them if they no longer have the capacity to do so themselves in the future—LPA in England and Wales or POA in Scotland.

- POA (Scotland):
  - A POA can deal with financial (FPA), property (PPA), and health/welfare matters (WPA).
  - Continuing FPA or PPA can come into effect whilst a person has capacity and will continue once they no longer have capacity.
  - WPA can only come into effect when the person lacks capacity.
  - If a POA is not appointed then the court can appoint a financial or welfare guardian.
- LPA (England and Wales)
  - An individual with capacity can appoint a LPA to make health decisions on their behalf if they lack capacity in the future.
  - The LPA must be registered with the Office of the Public Guardian.
  - The LPA must act according to the best interests of the individual.
  - Their jurisdiction only extends to decisions regarding life-sustaining treatment if this is expressly stated in the original application.
  - A valid ADRT drawn up after the appointment of an LPA must be honoured.

Case study

John was a 68-year-old man with a long history of chronic HF with severe LV systolic dysfunction due to ischaemic heart disease with previous MIs. Following his CABG 2yr previously, he had a secondary prevention CRTD inserted due to ventricular fibrillation (VF) following his operation. Unfortunately he went on to have multiple appropriate shocks from his defibrillator, requiring hospital admission. In addition he had AF, amiodarone-induced thyrotoxicosis, and problems with many HF medications due to significant symptomatic hypotension.

Understandably, after all his shocks from his device he became very anxious and at times quite agitated. He was, however, much calmer when with his family, especially his wife to whom he had been married for 25yr. With many alterations to his cardiac medications his rhythm became more stable and he stopped having multiple episodes of VT and shocks from his device. Although the shocks made him anxious he was keen to keep the device active while he felt well.

John deteriorated very quickly, but before this happened he had discussed with the cardiologist in the presence of his family what his wishes were including preferred place of care, preferred place of death, and resuscitation status. John did not want any further shocks from his device and when he deteriorated clinically arrangements were made for his device to be deactivated and an anticipatory care plan developed and communicated to all health care professionals involved in his care.

Within the anticipatory care plan there was clear guidance from the cardiologist about how to manage some the anticipated problems. As such with the support of the GP, district nurse, HF nurse and with a communication channel to the cardiologist John died comfortably at home and had no further hospital admissions.

Key components:

- Regular review by key worker to spot the clinical decline early.
- Open discussion surrounding end of life issues.
- Development of anticipatory care plan.
- Clear medical management guidance from cardiologist anticipating likely problems.
- Open channels of communication between primary and secondary care.
- Communication of document to all health professionals including OOH services.

Had John gone into hospital for whatever reason the anticipatory care document and medical management plan clearly stated that John was for palliative care, that he was not to be resuscitated, and that central IV lines, inotropes and referral to intensive care would not be appropriate.

When health care professionals do not know a patient, having clear guidance from the main care team which has been put in place with the patient and family allows them to follow the patient's wishes and ensure that the patient is comfortable, as such improving the quality of care in the dying phase for the patient and their family.

ACP and the medical management plan

- In ACP is important to ascertain and try to achieve the wishes of the patient. However, clear direction needs to be given by the medical team to all health professionals regarding the medical management of the patient.
- Whilst it is not possible to anticipate all eventualities, potential problems and their suggested management that can be foreseen should be documented.
- There should also be a clear line of communication for the GP and district nurse to obtain specialist advice if needed.
- For those patient who are admitted to hospital then the ceiling of appropriate medical therapy should be clearly documented and be accessible to all. Appropriate and clear planning can potentially prevent unnecessary and unwanted hospital admissions or facilitate early discharge.

Starting the conversation

Timing

- Doctors may feel nervous about starting the conversation, and patients may be waiting for the doctor to initiate this.
- Judging the timing of conversations, e.g. transition to end of life care, can be difficult in HF given the relapsing and remitting course.
- The question 'Is this patient at risk of dying in the next 6 to 12 months?' can help to identify those with whom to start the conversation about transition in goals of care and ACP leading towards end of life care.

Other possible triggers include:
- Disease progression, e.g. as assessed by NYHA class.
- Multiple hospital admissions, of increasing length.
- Deteriorating prognostic markers (see 📖 Chapter 3).
- Admission to a care home.

Skills required and content (see 📖 Chapter 4)

Adapting to the patient's pace, and maintenance of hope and optimism, are vital. A positive approach can be promoted by:
- Focusing on patient priorities now and for the future.
- Introduction of the concept of palliative care.
- A full holistic needs assessment.

Remember that:
- Communication is a *process*, not a single event.
- ACP is voluntary: no patient should be coerced into such discussions.

Further reading

Department of Health (2008) *End of life care strategy*, pp. 12, 17. Department of Health, London. Available at: http://www.cpa.org.uk/cpa/End_of_Life_Care_Strategy.pdf

General Medical Council (2008) *Consent: patients and doctors making decisions together*. General Medical Council, London. Available at: http://www.gmc-uk.org/guidance/ethical_guidance/consent_guidance_index.asp

General Medical Council (2010) *Treatment and care towards the end of life: good practice in decision making*. General Medical Council, London. Available at: http://www.gmc-uk.org/guidance/ethical_guidance/end_of_life_care.asp

Scottish Parliament (2000) *Adults with Incapacity Act*. Office of Public Sector Information, London. Available at: http://www.legislation.gov.uk/asp/2000/4/contents

References

1 Royal College of Physicians (2009) *Advance care planning.* Concise Guidance to Good Practice Series, No. 12. Royal College of Physicians, London
2 National End of Life Care Programme (2011) *Capacity, care planning and advance care planning in life limiting illness. A guide for health and social care staff.* Available at: http://www.endoflifecareforadults.nhs.uk/
3 UK Government (2005) *Mental Capacity Act.* Office of Public Sector Information, London. Available at: http://www.legislation.gov.uk/ukpga/2005/9/contents

Management of pain

Introduction

End-stage HF may not be thought of as a painful condition and therefore pain is an under-recognized symptom. The pain may be cardiac in origin or due to the comorbidities that many patients suffer. Untreated pain will further affect mobility thus aggravating other symptoms of breathlessness and fatigue made worse by cardiorespiratory conditioning and loss of skeletal muscle.

Prevalence of pain

A systematic review of studies of symptom prevalence consistently show that over half of patients with advanced HF report pain which may be severe and prolonged. This is consistent with the prevalence found in people with advanced malignancy, HIV disease, end-stage renal or respiratory disease.[1]

Impact

Comparison of the Edmonton Symptom Assessment Scale (ESAS) and Kansas City Cardiomyopathy Questionnaire (KCCQ) shows that general discomfort is one of the symptoms mostly related with the physical limitation domain of global health status. There did not appear to be an influence on the social functioning and the self-efficacy domains.[2] However, there is very little published work in this area.

Causes of pain

The common causes of pain in HF can be divided into cardiovascular, treatment-aggravated, and non-cardiovascular causes.

Cardiovascular

- Ischaemic chest pain (angina). Angina of effort may improve in end-stage disease as the patient is less active. Conversely it may be more problematic if the patient becomes too hypotensive to tolerate nitrate medication, or anaemia worsens their symptoms. If ischaemia is critical and results in unstable angina, this can cause difficulties with urgent OOH requests for analgesia resulting in inappropriate admissions to coronary care units.
- Ischaemic peripheral vascular disease (claudication/rest pain).
- Decubitus ulcers. Poor mobility and poor peripheral circulation, in conjunction with increased venous pressure leads to a high risk of ulceration. Poor healing and often comorbid diabetes aggravate this likelihood.
- Post-phlebitic syndrome (PPS). Patients with HF are at high risk of deep vein thrombosis (DVT). Pain is a common feature of PPS.

Treatment-aggravated

Diuretic therapy, especially loop diuretics, often needs to be adjusted in advanced HF. Diuretic therapy is associated with the following:
- Gout.
- Night cramps.

Non-cardiovascular

- Diabetic neuropathy (might strictly be classified as cardiovascular). In turn aggravates the risk of decubitus ulceration.
- Musculoskeletal.

Types of pain

For the purpose of management it is helpful to categorize pain into:
- Nociceptive.
- Neuropathic.
- Mixed nociceptive and neuropathic.
- Incident- or movement-related.

Nociceptive pain

Nociceptive pain, or the pain due to tissue damage, is usually responsive to opioid analgesia; the strength of analgesia needed will depend on the severity of the pain.

Neuropathic pain

Neuropathic pain usually has some opioid sensitivity. Adjuvant analgesics (see Chapter 9, Managing opioid side-effects, pp. 130–1) may be needed in addition to or instead of opioids if the dose of opioid required to relieve pain causes unacceptable side-effects.

Pain in people with HF may be a mixture of pain types: e.g. the pain of peripheral vascular disease is often due to tissue damage and inflammation, and neuropathic pain may be present if the peripheral nerves are also damaged. Therefore a mixture of types of analgesia may be required.

Incident or movement-related pain

This is usually caused by comorbid degenerative arthritis and can be more difficult to manage than other pain types. This is because pain may be controlled at rest but become very severe on movement, requiring high levels of analgesia. This could lead to unacceptable side-effects, particularly sleepiness, if given at times when the patient is at rest.

Other specific causes

It is important to diagnose other specific causes of pain as there may be specific remedies to relieve them.

Assessment of pain

- Pain is what the patient says it is.
- Pain is affected by all domains of life; physical, psychological, financial, and spiritual—so-called 'total pain' (Dame Cicely Saunders[3]).

A full assessment of the cause of the pain is key to an appropriate and effective management plan. As this must involve a discussion of all aspects of the pain, including its meaning (particularly pertinent to patients with angina) this assessment also often leads to the development of a good therapeutic relationship with the patient. It is also recognized that one of the most effective interventions for pain is the care and attention paid to the symptom by the clinician. Pain is usually not alleviated at the first attempt and a management plan must be closely monitored and the analgesics adjusted according to an individual's response (titration). This approach gives to the patient confidence in the clinician that also helps pain relief.

Areas covered by a pain assessment

- Site of pain.
- Duration of pain including whether it is:
  - constant,
  - intermittent,
  - day or night and whether it disturbs sleep.
- Provoking factors.
- Relieving factors.
- Radiation of pain.
- Intensity could be recorded as:
  - 'none', 'mild', 'moderate', or 'severe'; or
  - using a numerical rating scale 0–10 where 0 = no pain and 10 = pain as unbearable as you can imagine.
- Nature of pain, e.g. burning, stabbing.
- Presence of abnormal sensation.
- Mood (to exclude depression).
- Meaning of the pain to the individual.

Assessment tools

There are many pain assessment tools to choose from such as the McGill Pain Questionnaire and Brief Pain Inventory that were developed for use in cancer patients. Although not formerly validated in HF patients they are still likely to be useful. However, in regular clinical practice the use of a simple numerical rating scale, asking the patient to rate their severity of pain from 0 (no pain at all) through to 10 (the most severe pain imaginable) is easily used and can allow contemporaneous assessment of response to management. There are also simple clinical assessment mnemonics to help remember the aspects that need to be covered. A commonly used one is SOCRATES (Fig. 9.1).

S **Site of pain:** Where? Any radiation? Numbness where pain felt? Pattern of joint/muscle involvement?

O **Onset:** When did it start? How did it start? What started it? Change over time? History or injury?

C **Character of pain:** Type of pain — burning, shooting, stabbing, dull etc.

R **Radiation:** Does the pain go anywhere else?

A **Associated feature**

T **Timing/pattern:** Is it worse at any time of day? Is it associated with any particular activities?

E **Exacerbating and relieving factors**

S **Severity:** Record especially if the pain is chronic and you want to measure change over time, consider a patient diary. Ask about:
- Pain intensity e.g. none–mild–moderate–severe; rank on a 1–10 scale.
- Record interference with sleep or usual activities.
- Pain relief e.g. none–slight–moderate–good–complete.

Fig. 9.1 Example of a pain assessment system, SOCRATES. Reproduced from Watson, O'Reilly and Simon, 2010, *Pain and palliation*, p. 7 with permission of Oxford University Press.

What hinders pain management?

Clinical factors

A combination of clinician and patient factors contribute to poor pain recognition and management in this group of patients. Some of these are listed below.

Clinician factors

- Lack of recognition of the problem and therefore failure to assess in the clinic.
- Cause of pain not directly due to HF and therefore not seen as the role of the cardiologist to help it.
- Failure to monitor the effect of treatment and therefore adjust according to response.
- Fear of causing toxicity from opioids, especially a fear of respiratory depression which appears to be unfounded if carefully monitored.
- Fear of using strong opioids for non-cancer pain.
- Complex pain management because there is more than one cause of pain.
- Lack of recognition that established pain assessment and management tools have a place in HF leads to simple tools such as the World Health Organization (WHO) analgesic ladder not being applied. Therefore, patients may not be given NSAIDs for their gout as it is contra-indicated, but then receive nothing else in its place.

Patient factors

- Under-reporting of pain in the clinic.
- Cause of pain not directly due to heart disease and therefore not seen as the role of the cardiologist to help it.
- Analgesia not taken for fear of side-effects.
- Analgesia stopped because of side-effects but without request for review.
- Unfounded fear of addiction.
- Unfounded fear of tolerance and loss of effectiveness in the future 'when stronger pain killers might be needed'.

Drug handling in renal failure

Many patients with advanced HF also have renal dysfunction. Many drugs and their metabolites are excreted by the kidney through glomerular filtration, which, when reduced significantly, affects the clearance of those drugs and their metabolites. Where metabolites are active and retained, as is the case for morphine, the likelihood of toxicity is high.

Principles of management: the WHO analgesic ladder

Use of the WHO analgesic ladder (Fig. 9.2) to manage pain caused by cancer is recommended world-wide. Where pain is constant, as for much pain in people with HF, a similar method of pain control can be used with modifications to take account of the effect of poor renal function if present.

The principles are as follows:
- By mouth—where the patient can swallow and absorb.
- By the clock—if pain is constant, medication must be given regularly.
- By the ladder.
- With as needed (prn) medication if pain breaks through.
- For the individual.
- Attention to detail:
  - frequent assessment for efficacy and toxicity
  - dose adjustments according to assessment
  - aggressive management of side-effects.

Initial analgesia is selected according to the intensity of pain. When a numerical rating scale (NRS) of 0–10 is used, the following convention may be followed.
- Mild pain, scores 1–4: step 1 on the WHO analgesic ladder.
- Moderate pain, scores 5–6: step 2 on the WHO analgesic ladder.
- Severe pain, scores 7–10: step 3 on the WHO analgesic ladder.

At all stages appropriate adjuvant treatment can be added. If pain is not adequately controlled move up the ladder or, if already on step 3, the strong opioid is titrated upwards to pain relief.

Excellent SIGN guidelines for pain management for adults with cancer can be found at http://www.sign.ac.uk/pdf/SIGN106.pdf. Although drawn for cancer, the majority are applicable in HF apart from the exceptions highlighted in this section.

WHO analgesic ladder: steps 1 and 2

Step 1: non-opioids ± adjuvants
Paracetamol
- Metabolized by the liver; metabolites do occur but are accepted to be safe at the recommended dose of 1g four times a day (qds).

NSAIDs
- NSAIDS are contra-indicated in HF even in the presence of normal renal function because they cause retention of sodium and water which may precipitate cardiac decompensation and fluid overload.[4]

Step 2: opioids for mild to moderate pain + non-opioid ± adjuvants
Codeine
- Metabolized to codeine-6-glucurodine and morphine.
- Significant increase in half-life in renal failure.
- Accumulation of metabolites can cause drowsiness and confusion.

- Preparations combining codeine and paracetamol reduce the tablet burden.
- Preparations containing a codeine dose range from 8–30mg. The dose usually considered appropriate for mild to moderate pain is 60mg qds.
- Taking codeine and paracetamol together is more effective than codeine alone.

Tramadol
- Agonist at the μ opioid receptor.
- Metabolized in liver to O-desmethyltramadol.
- 90% excreted by kidney.
- 30% unchanged.
- Recommended dose for mild to moderate pain is 50mg qds.
- Accumulation will occur in renal impairment and the dose should be reduced and dose interval increased according to the degree of impairment.

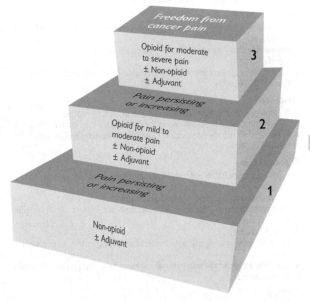

Fig. 9.2 The WHO analgesic ladder. Reproduced from http://www.who.int/cancer/palliative/painladder/en/ with permission of the World Health Association.

WHO analgesic ladder: step 3 opioids for moderate to severe pain + non-opioid ± adjuvant

All patients starting on strong opioids should be co-prescribed an anti-emetic and a laxative.

Morphine
- Metabolized to morphine-3-glucuronide (M3G) and morphine-6-glucuronide (M6G).
- M6G is a more potent analgesic than morphine.
- M3G and M6G accumulate in renal failure.
- Not recommended for chronic regular dosing in renal failure.
- Oral preparations include immediately available morphine, which should be given every 4hr (morphine sulphate solution, morphine tablets), or modified release (12-hourly preparations or 24-hourly preparations).
- In the absence of renal failure, morphine should be the strong opioid of first choice as it is widely available in a variety of preparations and the majority of doctors should be familiar with its use.

Hydromorphone
- Synthetic μ agonist; when used orally 4–7 times as potent as oral morphine.
- Metabolized to hydromorphone-3-glucuronide (H3G) and other metabolites.
- Preparations include immediately available (4-hourly) and modified release (12-hourly).

Oxycodone
- A semi-synthetic μ agonist with a similar profile to morphine.
- 90% of the drug is metabolized in the liver with active metabolites.
- Preparations include immediately available (4-hourly) and modified release (12-hourly).

Buprenorphine
- A partial μ agonist/antagonist; SL 30–60 times as potent as oral morphine.
- Metabolized to buprenorphine-3-glucuronide (B3G). and norbuprenorphine (NorB) in the liver. Both accumulate significantly in renal failure.
- B3G is inactive.
- NorB has minor analgesic activity and causes respiratory depression in rats.
- Considered generally safe in renal impairment as the pharmacokinetics are unaltered.

Fentanyl
- Potent synthetic μ agonist 50–100 times as potent as morphine.
- 1000 times as lipophilic as morphine and therefore suitable for transdermal (TD) administration.
- Available as buccal or SL tablets and nasal spray preparations for quick-onset analgesia (only for patients already on regular doses of strong opioids of 40mg morphine equivalent doses/24hr).

- Metabolized in the liver to norfentanyl, which is inactive; therefore accumulation is not clinically important.
- <10% excreted unchanged in the urine.
- Safe opioid for SC infusion at the end of life if there is renal failure.
- Preferred opioid for titration using prn SC administration at end of life if there is renal failure, even if alfentanil is in the syringe driver as it has a longer duration of action than alfenantil.
- TD fentanyl can be used for *stable*, *continuous* pain in HF once the patient's opioid requirement has been titrated with an immediately available preparation.

NB: Although TD fentanyl should not be used for uncontrolled or unstable pain, in the event of a patient who is already stabilized on TD fentanyl developing escalating or unpredictable pain, the TD fentanyl patch should remain at the same dose and any additional requirement titrated using an immediately available opioid preparation such as oral morphine sulphate solution in the appropriate breakthrough pain dose. Discussion with the pharmacist or palliative care team is advised.

Important considerations when using TD fentanyl
- Not appropriate for uncontrolled pain.
- Effective analgesia not reached until 24hr after the patch is applied.
- When starting the first patch continue normal release medications for the first 12hr and ensure the patient knows that further doses may be needed while the dose of fentanyl from the patch builds up in the blood.
- A normal release strong opioid such as morphine must be available for breakthrough pain.
- Maximum analgesia may not be reached until 72hr so the patch dose should not be increased until it is time for a patch change.
- A depot of fentanyl remains under the skin for 24hr after patch removal.
- If naloxone is needed to reverse narcosis a 24hr infusion may be needed.
- If pain is relieved by another means, such as a nerve block or palliative radiotherapy, it is important to remember the potential for toxicity from prolonged action of fentanyl.
- Patients should be monitored closely. In theory it might be expected that the dose could gradually be reduced, though there is no evidence from practice.

Alfentanil
- A derivative of fentanyl.
- It is one-quarter to one-fifth as potent as fentanyl but approximately 10 times more potent than SC diamorphine or 15 times as potent as SC morphine.
- It is extensively metabolized in the liver with inactive metabolites.
- Useful for continuous SC infusions because of greater solubility than fentanyl.
- It has a short duration of action when given SC so is not useful for titrating opioid against pain relief (use fentanyl).
- It is useful for short episodes of predictable pain, e.g. procedure-related pain.

Methadone
- Synthetic opioid active at μ opioid receptor.
- Thought to have some activity as a *N*-methyl-D-aspartate (NMDA) receptor antagonist and therefore a possible role in neuropathic pain.
- It is excreted mainly in the faeces, but is also metabolized in the liver to inactive metabolites.
- In the anuric patient excretion is almost exclusively faecal.
- Methadone titration for pain relief needs specialist experience because of its prolonged pharmacological action—up to 60hr—and individual pharmacokinetics.

Parenteral opioids
- Preferred route is SC.
- If normal or mild renal dysfunction, the preferred strong opioids for continuous infusion are diamorphine or morphine. The equivalent 24hr dose is approximately one-third of the 24hr oral morphine dose. The prn dose should be one-sixth of the 24hr dose.
- In renal failure, the preferred strong opioid for titrating and breakthrough pain is fentanyl: suggested doses 12.5–25mcg SC prn hourly (titrate to higher dose if needed); for doses greater than 600mcg/24hr use alfentanil.

Recommendations
In a patient with normal renal function and who has been taking two tablets of co-codamol (paracetamol 500mg/codeine 30mg) qds, start with 10mg of immediately available oral morphine solution or tablets. However, this dose may need to be reduced to 5mg if the patient has been taking a lower dose of codeine (or none), or weighs less than 60 kg. Allow additional prn medication if the pain is not controlled. When the 24hr dose is stable, convert to a modified-release preparation (i.e. if pain is controlled with 60mg morphine, change to 30mg bd of modified-release morphine). prn medication should be available as immediately available morphine at a dose of one-sixth of the 24hr dose.

In severe renal dysfunction (creatinine clearance, CrCL, <30ml/min) the preferred strong opioids are: fentanyl, alfentanil, or buprenorphine.

Summary of the WHO analgesic ladder

General points
- Assess the patient's pain.
- Choose the appropriate step.
- Give drug regularly plus prn for breakthrough pain or incident pain.
- Monitor for toxicity and efficacy.
- Adjust and move up a step or increase dose as needed.
- Remember psychological, social, and spiritual distress will impact on pain.

Step 1
- Non-opioid ± adjuvants. Paracetamol 1g qds ± adjuvants if safe and indicated.

Step 2
- Non-opioid +opioid for mild-moderate pain ± adjuvant.
- Paracetamol 1g + codeine 60mg qds (can prescribe in combined preparation).

OR
- Paracetamol 1g + tramadol 50mg qds + adjuvants if safe and indicated.

Step 3
- Non-opioid + opioid for moderate to severe pain + adjuvants.

If the patient is able to swallow oral medication:
- Paracetamol 1g qds +
  - Morphine 5–10mg every 4hr and prn for breakthrough pain.
  - When pain is controlled, calculate the total daily dose of morphine and administer as bd modified-release preparation providing the same total daily dose.
  - Allow prn medication using immediately available morphine at one-sixth the total daily dose of morphine.
  - Regular review is required to assess whether this dose is appropriate.
  - ± adjuvants if safe and indicated.

Patient unable to swallow oral medication:
- If normal renal function:
  - If opioid naïve, start with diamorphine 10mg/24hr by continuous SC infusion and allow 2.5mg prn for breakthrough pain.
  - If already on opioids, then the 24hr dose of diamorphine is approximately one-third of the previous 24hr dose of oral morphine, plus allow a dose of approximately one-sixth total daily dose as prn.

If renal failure (CrCL <30ml/min)
- If opioid naïve, start with 12.5–25mcg fentanyl available up to hourly. After 24hr, calculate the total 24hr dose required for analgesia and administer via continuous SC infusion.
- If on opioids, then dose for continuous SC infusion will depend on previous requirements, converting to a dose equivalent.

Managing opioid side-effects

Many of the unwanted effects from opioids can be predicted and the very common ones such as nausea/vomiting and constipation should be anticipated by co-prescription of anti-emetics and laxatives. Some are less common, but should be noticed and managed appropriately by regular review of the patient. As renal dysfunction is common in end-stage HF, especial care should be taken if a patient is on an opioid known to accumulate in renal failure. Many unwanted effects mimic signs and symptoms of uraemia and a proper assessment should be made. If renal failure has developed, then the opioid should be changed to fentanyl or alfentanil as described in 📖 Chapter 9, Principles of management: the WHO analgesic ladder, pp. 125–9.

Opioid toxicity may occur if too rapid a dose titration has been attempted.

The development of opioid toxicity in a patient who has had no problem on a stable dose of opioid usually signals a change in clinical situation such as:

- Development or worsening of renal dysfunction.
- MI.
- Infection.
- Dehydration (including over-diuresis).

General approach

- Assess for reversible precipitants as above and treat.
- Most side-effects settle after a few days after starting or increasing the dose.
- If symptoms persist despite appropriate measures, reduce the dose of opioid by approximately one-third and attempt titration again, but at a slower rate.
- If symptoms persist, then a switch to another opioid, or a non-opioid method of pain control may be required.
- If switching to a different opioid, discussion with the specialist palliative care team is advised.

Opioid side-effects

Gastrointestinal effects
Nausea and vomiting

- Occur in approximately a quarter of patients.
- Wear off after 10–14 days.
- Make anti-emetic available when starting opioids (see 📖 Chapter 10, Other symptoms, pp. 146–8).

Constipation

- Nearly universal.
- Provide all patients with laxatives (see 📖 Chapter 10, Other symptoms, pp. 146–8).

Central nervous system (CNS) effects
Drowsiness

- More common when first starting opioid or increasing the dose.
- May reduce after 72hr.

- If it continues consider an alternative opioid or alternative means of pain control.

Confusion
- Occurrence as for drowsiness.
- Exclude correctable causes.
- Reduce dose.
- Consider an alternative opioid or means of pain relief.

Other CNS effects
- Myoclonic jerks

Respiratory depression

Respiratory depression is *not* a problem *if*:
- Opioids dose is titrated upwards against pain because patients become tolerant to the respiratory depressant effect.
- Short-acting preparations are used for titration.
- Dose titration takes place prior to placement of a fentanyl patch.
- Pain is suddenly relieved by a procedure such as nerve block and systemic analgesia is stopped and re-titrated.

Respiratory depression *can* occur, however:
- When the clinical situation changes.
- When pain is reduced but analgesia is not.
- If the patient not carefully monitored.

Adjuvant analgesia

Adjuvant analgesics are drugs which have a primary purpose other than analgesia but which may be useful in specific clinical situations to help relieve pain. They can be used in addition to opioids and may help reduce the dose of opioid required.

Pain syndromes

Neuropathic pain

Some pain in HF is neuropathic, e.g. due to co-morbid diabetic neuropathy or nerve root pain resulting from degenerative arthritis of the spine.

The two main classes of drug used as adjuvant analgesics are tricyclic antidepressants and anticonvulsants.

Antidepressants
- Tricyclic antidepressants are anticholinergic and therefore should be avoided in HF as they are pro-arrhythmic.
- Newer antidepressants such as mirtazapine (a pre-synaptic alpha-adrenoceptor antagonist), and venlafaxine (a serotonin and norepinephrine re-uptake inhibitor) have been reported to be helpful in neuropathic pain and appear to be cardiac safe.
- Concerns over venlafaxine seem to have been unfounded.
- Titration should start using the lowest dose available, and analgesia is usually achieved with doses much lower than those needed for depression.

Anticonvulsants
The two most commonly used anticonvulsants are gabapentin and pre-gabalin:
- There are some case reports of pregabalin exacerbating HF, but gabapentin appears to be cardiac safe.
- Sedation is often a problem during initial titration especially in frail elderly patients with comorbidities, and thus a slow titration starting at 100–300mg nocte, aiming for a daily dose of 900–2400mg prn and as tolerated.
- Gabapentin doses must be reduced in renal failure.

Carbamazepine is another recognized neuropathic adjuvant anticonvulsant. However, it has a narrow therapeutic window, has several drug interactions and can be difficult for the patient to manage amongst their multidrug regimen.

Gout

Gout is common and debilitating and is often precipitated by alteration in the diuretic regime.
- NSAIDs are contra-indicated.
- Treat the acute attack with colchicine; 500mcg 2–4 times daily until symptoms resolve (maximum dose per course 6mg, do not repeat the course within 3 days).
- If colchicine not tolerated, treat with low dose (10mg per day) of prednisolone until symptoms settle.
- Once acute symptoms settle, the patient should be treated with long prophylaxis with allopurinol 100–300mg per day started 1–2 weeks after the acute attack.

Topical methods of analgesia

Opioids

Opioids may be effective topically where the skin is broken and there is inflammation as opioid receptors migrate to areas of inflammation. Most experience relates to morphine in a hydrogel such as Intrasite® gel, though other opioids such as fentanyl and diamorphine have been used. As the effect is local and relatively low doses are used it is thought that there is little effect from systemic absorption.

Indications
- Ischaemic leg ulcer that is painful between dressing changes.
- Decubitus ulcer for which treatment is palliative and healing is not expected.

Possible prescription
- Morphine (for injection) 10mg in Intrasite® gel applied to the ulcer daily.

Capsaicin cream

Capsaicin is a chilli alkaloid that depletes substance P. There is evidence for benefit when it is used for post-herpetic neuralgia, diabetic neuropathy, and osteoarthritis though a significant proportion of people will not tolerate it as it causes burning prior to relief.

Possible uses:
- Localized areas of neuropathic pain from diabetic neuropathy (number needed to treat (NNT) = 4).
- Osteoarthritis (NNT = 3).

Topical NSAIDs

These may be useful for localized joint pain with non-ulcerated skin. (NNT = 3). Systemic NSAIDs are contra-indicated.

Episodic, movement related, or incident pain

Pain may still occur despite being well controlled for most of the time. Careful review should ensure this is not just due to 'end of dose failure' due to insufficient dose of modified-release 12-hourly morphine. Episodic pain may be spontaneous or precipitated by a predictable incident such as moving, or having a painful procedure such as a change of a leg ulcer dressing. Careful assessment and management is required, or opioid toxicity may be precipitated by inappropriate upwards titration of background modified-release opioid dose.

These pains can be divided into the following categories.

Spontaneous episodes of pain
- Usually neuropathic.
- May be short-lived but severe.
- Shooting or burning in nature.
- No precipitating factors.
- Consider neuropathic agent for pain relief.

Breakthrough pain occurring during dose titration
- Background analgesia inadequate.
- Occurs at end of a dosing period indicating a higher dose is needed.
- Explain to patient and continue dose titration.

Dose of breakthrough medication related to the 24hr opioid taken
- For hydromorphone, morphine, and oxycodone: one-sixth of the 24hr dose.
- For fentanyl and alfentanil: one-tenth of the 24hr dose titrating up to one-sixth if ineffective.

Movement-related or incident pain
- Patient pain-free at rest but severe pain on movement or dressing change.
- Gradually titrate background opioid to highest level tolerated by the patient.
- Use short-acting opioid prior to planned activity, e.g. dressing change. Choose drug and route depending on patient's condition and length of procedure:
  - oral hydromorphone: onset 30min, duration 4hr
  - SC fentanyl: onset 5–10min, duration 1–2hr
  - SC alfentanil: onset 3–5min, duration about 30–60min
  - buccal/nasal/SL alfentanil: onset 5–10min, duration 20min.
- Entonox® (inhaled nitrous oxide) may have a role for episodes of care in those who are not too frail.
- Look for local means of relieving pain, e.g. joint immobilization.
- Consider nerve blocks or anaesthetic procedure.

Buccal, SL, and nasal fentanyl
For patients established on at least 40mg oral morphine equivalent, there are now preparations for transmucosal delivery of fentanyl, if an opioid

with an onset of action as quick as alfentanil, but with a longer duration of action, is required. Discussion with the specialist palliative care team is recommended.

Buccal, nasal, or SL alfentanil

Reasonable bioavailability and good solubility mean that a sufficient dose of alfentanil can be given buccally to achieve short-term (15–20min) analgesia to cover painful procedures or planned painful activities. The provision of metered dosing delivering 0.14mL (0.14mg) per spray enables the patient to have control. Alfentanil has approximately one-fifth the potency of fentanyl;[5] thus the dose delivered is approximately equivalent to 15–30mcg of fentanyl. The dose required will vary from patient to patient, but it is reasonable to start with three sprays, which delivers a dose of 0.42mg, increasing the number of sprays if needed. Doses greater than 1.5mL are likely to be swallowed rather than absorbed buccally so are unlikely to be effective.[5]

NB: This use of alfentanil is an off-label use of the drug and should be monitored. Discussion with the specialist palliative care team is recommended.

Chronic pain clinic referral and anaesthetic procedures

In some situations management of severe chronic pain can be exceedingly difficult and the patient may be helped by referral to a chronic pain management team where they may benefit from management by the multidisciplinary pain team.

Anaesthetic procedures may be indicated in some of the following situations:

- Severe neuropathic pain where spinal analgesia could be an option.
- Incident pain, such as that from a fractured hip where the patient is not fit for surgery, for local anaesthetic block.
- Sympathetically mediated pain.
- Difficulty in achieving satisfactory pain control despite escalating analgesia or because of unacceptable toxicity when analgesia is achieved.

Unremitting angina

- Occasionally a patient with unremitting angina may need referral for spinal cord stimulation.
- Acupuncture may also be helpful.
- These procedures are contra-indicated in the presence of pacemaker devices.

Referral to the palliative care team

When pain is difficult to manage or there are other distressing symptoms or psychological or social issues, referral to your local palliative care team may give the opportunity for a holistic assessment and review with improvement in symptoms. The presence of severe pain as part of disease progression and patient deterioration often indicates that prognosis is reduced or short. It should therefore act as a trigger for referral to a palliative care service. This can occur even if prognosis is uncertain, as good symptom relief and support should improve the patient's quality of life. It may also enable discussions about future care to be started. See also ☐ Chapter 6.

References

1 Solano JP, Gomes B, Higginson IJ (2006) A comparison of symptom prevalence in far advanced cancer, AIDS, heart disease, chronic obstructive pulmonary disease and renal disease. *J Pain Symptom Manage* **31**, 58–69.
2 Opasich C, Gualco A, De FS et al. (2008) Physical and emotional symptom burden of patients with end-stage heart failure: what to measure, how and why. *J Cardiovasc Med* **9**, 1104–8.
3 Saunders CM (1978) *The management of terminal disease*. Edward Arnold, London.
4 Heerdink ER, Leufkens HG, Herings RM, Ottervanger JP, Stricker BH, Bakker A (1998) NSAIDs associated with increased risk of congestive heart failure in elderly patients taking diuretics. *Arch Intern Med* **158**, 1108–12.
5 Twycross R, Wilcock A (2007) *The palliative care formulary*, 3rd edn (PCF3). Radcliffe Medical Press, Oxford.

Symptoms other than pain

Introduction

Although palliative care services in the UK have grown up around cancer services, three-quarters of deaths in the developed world are due to non-cancer diseases including HF. As long ago as 1963, Hinton observed that patients dying from heart or renal failure seemed to have more physical and mental distress than those dying from cancer.[1] A systematic review of 64 papers assessing symptom burden in cancer, HIV, renal disease, HF, and respiratory disease found very little difference in the symptom burden of 11 common symptoms (Table 10.1 shows figures for cancer and heart disease), but it is only relatively recently that those due to non-cancer diseases are being actively addressed.[2] Even if physical problems might be given some attention, a holistic approach assessing all aspects of the symptoms (psychological, social, financial, and spiritual support) is often less forthcoming for the patient with HF than for the patient with cancer.[3]

Principles of symptom control

- All patients should have a comprehensive assessment including thorough history, examination, and relevant investigations.
- The assessment is part of a global assessment of physical, psychological, social, and spiritual need.
- Cardiac treatments are integral to good symptom control and should be optimized according to patient tolerance.
- The core management plan should include explanation and discussion.
- Reversible causes of symptoms should be treated wherever possible.
- Treatment should be reviewed regularly.

Key symptoms in HF

- The cardinal symptoms of breathlessness and fatigue help form the NYHA classification of HF (see Table 2.1).
- Patients with end-stage disease will have NYHA III (comfortable at rest but marked limitation of physical activity) or NYHA IV (symptomatic at rest and unable to carry out physical activity without more discomfort) disease.

Table 10.1 Cancer and heart disease symptoms compared

Symptom	Cancer	Heart disease
Pain	35–96%	41–77%
Depression	3–77%	9–36%
Anxiety	13–79%	49%
Confusion	6–93%	18–32%
Fatigue	32–90%	69–82%
Breathlessness	10–70%	60–88%
Insomnia	9–69%	36–48%
Nausea	6–68%	17–48%
Constipation	23–65%	38–42%
Diarrhoea	3–29%	12%
Anorexia	30–92%	21–41%

Reprinted from Solano JP, Gomes B, Higginson IJ, A comparison of symptom prevalence in far advanced cancer, AIDS, heart disease, chronic obstructive pulmonary disease and renal disease, *Journal of Pain Symptom Management*, Volume 31, Issue 1, pp. 58–69, 2006 with permission from Elsevier.

Breathlessness

Breathlessness is frightening to both patients and those caring for them. It is closely related to anxiety and panic, and can be particularly concerning at night if nocturnal breathlessness is a problem.

Management of breathlessness is of key importance, as not only is it a cause of distress to the patient and their family but it is also associated with a high risk of inappropriate hospital admission.

Assessment should look for potentially reversible or other causes of breathlessness:

• Fluid overload requiring optimization of diuretics.
• Infection.
• Pulmonary emboli.
• Optimal treatment of comorbidities such as asthma and chronic obstructive pulmonary disease (COPD).
• Cardiorespiratory de-conditioning.
• Lung neoplasm.
• Respiratory disease such as COPD, pulmonary fibrosis, bronchiectasis, etc.
• Arrhythmias such as atrial fibrillation with a fast ventricular rate.

No apparent cause of breathlessness may be found. This is because patients with HF have increased chemoceptor sensitivity and an increased muscle ergoreflex response to exercise. The pattern of respiration and lung perfusion/ventilation is inefficient, resulting in increased physical and physiological dead space.[4]

Management should include both non-pharmacological and pharmacological interventions.

Non-pharmacological interventions[5]

These should be the mainstay of treatment and started as early as possible. Involvement of the multiprofessional team, including physiotherapy and occupational therapy, are therefore crucial:

• Exercise. Even patients who are unwell should be encouraged to exercise within their limitations, as anything that helps preserve muscle bulk will help breathlessness. Advice should be sought from experienced physiotherapists.
• Pacing and prioritizing, including provision of home aids to daily living.
• Anxiety/panic management.
• Breathing exercises to retrain inefficient patterns of ventilation.
• Use of a hand-held fan. The passage of cool air across the lower face (innervated by the 2nd and 3rd branches of the trigeminal nerve) can be helpful and should be tried before oxygen, unless there is another indication for oxygen such as hypoxic confusion.
• Use of mobility aids such as walking sticks and wheeled walkers.

Pharmacological interventions

Oxygen

- Oxygen would seem an obvious choice to alleviate breathlessness, but patients with compensated HF tend not to desaturate and it does not appear to be of benefit unless there are other factors causing hypoxia.[6–8]
- Individual assessment should be made rather than an automatic use of expensive and potentially intrusive treatment inducing psychological dependence.
- If nocturnal central apnoea is a problem leading to daytime somnolence and morning headache, nocturnal oxygen may be helpful.

Opioids

- There is evidence from studies in patients with intractable breathlessness from any cause that low-dose opioids confer a small but clinically significant benefit.[9,10]
- There is conflicting evidence with regard to opioid use in HF.[11,12] Therefore a therapeutic trial with a clear review to see if the patient has benefited or not is important.
- Oral morphine 2.5–5mg qds appears to be tolerated well in patients with adequate renal function (CrCL> 30 ml/min).
- Patients with advanced disease may experience periodic ventilation with central apnoea. Opioids may help this, and if the patient is unable to swallow oral morphine, it could be administered as 5–10mg diamorphine or morphine/24hr via syringe driver, or 0.5–1mg alfentanil/24hr if there is renal dysfunction.

Benzodiazepines

- Anxiety and panic are often part of the experience of breathlessness.
- Regular administration of benzodiazepines should be avoided because of the risk of falls and memory loss.
- Shorter-duration, quicker onset-of-action preparations such as SL lorazepam 0.5–1mg prn for panic may be useful.
- If anxiety appears to be persistent, then the use of an anxiolytic antidepressant such as mirtazepine would be preferable to regular benzodiazepines.

If breathlessness is distressing in the dying patient, then sedation with midazolam, starting at 10mg/24hr via a syringe driver and titrated daily to effect using prn doses of 2.5–5mg may be needed. Patients are often frightened of dying with breathlessness and can be reassured that sedation may be used if that is their wish.

Other symptoms

Fatigue

Potentially reversible factors include:
- Hypokalaemia from loop diuretics.
- Overdiuresis.
- Anaemia.
- Beta-blockers; balance of benefit/burden to be weighed.
- Insomnia.
- Depression.

Management
- Drug related: depending on the role of beta-blockers in the patient, the dose may need to be reduced or even stopped, particularly if symptomatic bradycardia or hypotension persist. Nocturnal dosing may allow the drug to be continued.
- Anaemia: a further assessment of the cause is required—may be iron deficient due to aspirin therapy, or anaemia of chronic disease/renal disease. If chronic disease/renal disease then iron infusion ± erythropoietin may be indicated.
- Insomnia: a further assessment of cause required—may be sleep apnoea (trial of opioids or oxygen or non-invasive nocturnal ventilation); paroxysmal nocturnal dyspnoea/orthopnoea (optimize fluid balance and provide a back raiser or even hospital bed); nocturnal pain (see Chapter 9); anxiety/depression (see Chapter 11). Amitriptyline should be avoided as a night sedative because of its anticholinergic effects.

In general
- Pacing: prioritizing of activities to minimize fatigue.
- Energy-saving aids.
- Exercise within limitations, aiming to maintain muscle bulk and cardiorespiratory conditioning.

Nausea and anorexia

Patients become cachectic in the end stage of heart disease due to the negative effect of the neuroendocrine response on metabolism and appetite.[13] However, a full nutritional assessment to exclude reversible causes of weight loss is important as a decrease in intake, although not the trigger for cachexia, may contribute to its progression. Diuretics may lead to loss of micronutrients and gut oedema may affect absorption.

General causes of problems with eating:
- Fatigue after food preparation, which maybe alleviated by assistance with meals/shopping, etc.
- Breathlessness affecting eating.
- Oral candidiasis.
- Ill-fitting dentures.
- Change in taste, sometimes due to medication.
- Dry mouth from mouth breathing or diuretics.

Causes of nausea include:
- Liver congestion from fluid overload.
- Gut wall congestion from fluid overload, which may in turn affect nutritional status.
- Cardiac medication: spironolactone, aspirin, digoxin toxicity, or simply because of polypharmacy.
- Medication for comorbidities: antibiotics, metformin, theophylline toxicity.
- Medication for pain or breathlessness: opioids.
- Constipation.
- Renal failure.
- Anxiety.
- Cooking smells which may be offputting.

Anti-emetic choice
- Prokinetics such as metoclopramide 10mg tds–qds or domperidone 10mg tds–qds are well tolerated. Metoclopramide should be avoided if there is comorbid Parkinsonism.
- Haloperidol and levomepromazine are also well tolerated and will not increase bowel activity. However, the dose should be kept low (haloperidol 0.5–1.5mg daily, levomepromazine 6mg bd) to minimize the risk of unwanted sedation and hypotension. Avoid in Parkinsonism unless in the dying phase.
- Cyclizine should be avoided except in the dying phase because it is anticholinergic.
- Anti-emetics should be prescribed and reviewed regularly.

Skin care and itch
- This is important because of recurrent problems with peripheral oedema, poor mobility, and poor peripheral circulation, all of which increase the risk of cellulitis and ulceration.
- Daily application of emollients such as aqueous cream is helpful. If itch is present this can be prepared with 1% menthol.
- Keeping emollients in the fridge is a useful tip.
- Itch may be a problem because of the thinning skin of old age and be exacerbated by the presence of renal dysfunction.
- Selective serotonin re-uptake inhibitors/serotonin–norepinephrine re-uptake inhibitors (SSRIs/SNRIs) such as paroxetine (20mg daily) or mirtazapine (15mg nocte) may ease itch.
- Sedating antihistamines are disappointing, although if used at night may help sleep.
- Other drugs such as ondansetron and thalidomide may be used off-licence, but there is only a small evidence base to support their use and should be reserved for intractable itch. Discussion with the palliative care team is advised.

Constipation
- Constipation is common, neglected, and debilitating, uses valuable and scarce energy, and exacerbates breathlessness, nausea, anorexia, and pain.

- Avoid bulk-forming agents such as ispaghula husk in patients on fluid restriction unless there is a specific indication such as diarrhoea from diverticular disease or irritable bowel disease.
- Use a softening agent such as lactulose or polymacrogols (e.g. Movicol®—there is some sodium in the preparation, but it is unlikely to be clinically significant). Laxatives should be titrated to effect and taken regularly to prevent swinging from diarrhoea to constipation.

When to involve the palliative care team

Symptoms may be straightforward to ease, but where they are persistent or complex, particularly when aggravated by psychological or existential distress, liaison with the palliative care team is recommended.

References

1 Hinton JM (1963) The physical and mental distress of the dying. *Q J Med* **32**, 1–21.
2 Solano JP, Gomes B, Higginson IJ (2006) A comparison of symptom prevalence in far advanced cancer, AIDS, heart disease, chronic obstructive pulmonary disease and renal disease. *J Pain Symptom Manage* **31**, 58–69.
3 Anderson H, Ward C, Eardley A et al. (2001) The concerns of patients under palliative care and a heart failure clinic are not being met. *Palliat Med* **15**, 279–86.
4 Clark AL, McDonagh T (1997) The origin of symptoms in chronic heart failure. *Heart* **78**, 429–30.
5 Bausewein C, Booth S, Gysels M, Higginson I (2008) Non-pharmacological interventions for breathlessness in advanced stages of malignant and non-malignant diseases. *Cochrane Database Syst Rev* **2008**(2), CD005623.
6 Currow DC, McDonald CF, Frith PA et al. (2010) Effect of palliative oxygen versus room air in relief of breathlessness in patients with refractory dyspnoea: a double-blind, randomised controlled trial. *Lancet* **376**, 784–93.
7 Currow DC, Agar M, Smith J, Abernethy AP (2009) Does palliative home oxygen improve dyspnoea? A consecutive cohort study. *Palliat Med* **23**, 309–16.
8 Clark AL, Johnson MJ, Squire I (2011) Does home oxygen benefit people with chronic heart failure? *BMJ* **342**, d234.
9 Jennings AL, Davies AN, Higgins JP, Gibbs JS, Broadley KE (2002) A systematic review of the use of opioids in the management of dyspnoea. *Thorax* **57**, 939–44.
10 Abernethy AP, Currow DC, Frith P, Fazekas BS, McHugh A, Bui C (2003) Randomised, double blind, placebo controlled crossover trial of sustained release morphine for the management of refractory dyspnoea. *BMJ* **327**, 523–8.
11 Johnson MJ, McDonagh TA, Harkness A, McKay SE, Dargie HJ (2002) Morphine for the relief of breathlessness in patients with chronic heart failure—a pilot study. *Eur J Heart Fail* **4**, 753–6.
12 Oxberry SG, Torgerson DJ, Bland JM, Clark AL, Cleland JGF, Johnson MJ (2011) Short-term opioids for breathlessness in stable chronic heart failure: a randomized controlled trial. *Eur J Heart Fail* **13**, 1006–12.
13 von HS, Lainscak M, Springer J, Anker SD (2009) Cardiac cachexia: a systematic overview. *Pharmacol Ther* **121**, 227–52.

Psychological and psychosocial aspects of HF

Introduction

Psychological problems are common in chronic illness, and it is well recognized that depression, for example, is more common in people with concurrent physical diseases than in the general population.

Patients with HF have to cope with progressive debilitation, lessening ability, and increasing dependence upon others. In effect, these sequential losses are like repeated bereavements, and whilst most people cope with most things most of the time using ways of coping that have stood them in good stead over the years, others fail to adjust, or find that their previous ways of dealing with difficult circumstances are now less robust, and anxiety and depression may ensue.

Social issues also cause much difficulty in the last stage of a patient's life and can have a big impact on whether someone is able to be cared for and die in their own home. The 'end of life' in HF can last for months, if not longer, and attention to this aspect is crucial but often overlooked.

Coping

- Most people cope with most things most of the time without recourse to the help of health care professionals.
- Most people, if they do need the help of health care professionals, will benefit from the support and skills of the GP, HF nurse, cardiologist, or palliative physician.
- A few will need the experience and training of clinical psychologists and psychiatrists, and identifying this particular group is a key skill.

An understanding of how a patient has coped over the years can often be gained simply by asking questions such as 'What are your strengths?' and 'How have you coped with hard times in the past?'. Such probing is also useful in helping the patient regain a sense of self where this has been lost and lead to joint decision-making where this is something the patient wishes.

Engaging with decisions as a way of coping

It is important to understand that some patients find it helpful to be involved in decisions about their management whereas others do not. It is necessary to address each person individually without making any assumption as to how they cope, or are able to handle information. A failure to do this, i.e. by giving too much or too little information, may precipitate or aggravate psychological distress, especially towards the end of life when patients may not have the capacity or flexibility to use any coping strategy other than those which have served them in the past.

Coping strategies for living with HF

Living with progressive disease is a difficult balance of accepting the reality of increasing disability and life-limiting illness whilst retaining the ability to enjoy life. Well-recognized patient strategies to try to live with this paradox include:
- Avoidance (active avoidance of unfavourable information).
- Disavowal (while understanding the seriousness of the situation dissociating this unconsciously from personal reality).
- Acceptance (conscious acceptance using understanding and control).[1]
- Combinations of the above.

In Buetow et al.'s large and representative study,[1] no patient demonstrated outright denial, but nearly all found some way to downplay the situation in order to maintain hope. Any communication of diagnosis and prognosis, therefore, has to be done gently, as many will find this difficult, if it does not 'fit' with the way they are coping with their illness.

When communication fails or is bad

- If difficult conversations are avoided the patient is denied possible assistance, support, and opportunities to be involved in their end of life care.
- If difficult conversations are handled badly and insensitively without an awareness of how the patient may be dealing with their illness, they could be 'pushed' into an anxiety state or depression.

Depression

Depression is:
- Common in patients with HF; prevalence estimates range between 24% and 42%.[2]
- Often goes undiagnosed and untreated; dismissed as 'understandable'.
- Difficult to recognize as many of the symptoms mimic those of the underlying physical illness, particularly in advanced disease.
- Independently associated with repeat hospital admissions.
- Independently associated with a worse prognosis.
- Associated with poor social support, which in turn is associated with a poorer outcome in HF.
- Affects compliance with drug and exercise treatments.

Depression in HF responds to standard treatments for depression, although we do not know yet whether this has any impact on the hospital admission or mortality outcomes associated with depression.

Patients who are in the last few days of life will not have time to respond to drug therapy for depression. However, people with advanced HF may often really benefit from active treatment of their depression even if they are in the last few months of life. Successful treatment will help them:
- Take part in important discussions with regard to their place of care.
- Put their affairs in order.
- Leave their loved ones with memories that are much more helpful in bereavement than those provided by a patient who has been depressed for the last few months of life.

Screening for depression

The benefits of routinely screening the general population for depression has been brought into question. However, screening in high risk populations, such as those with chronic illness, especially when the screening is part of an overall structure of care designed to fully assess and manage psychological concerns,[3] is more likely to be beneficial.

In practice two simple questions can be asked to see whether a more in-depth assessment is needed:
- 'Have you felt depressed or low in mood every day for the past two weeks?'.
- 'Can you still find pleasure in life?'.

Treatment for depression

Treatment can be pharmacological or non-pharmacological.

Non-pharmacological
- Exercise programmes within the patient's limitations may be helpful.
- Cognitive behavioural therapies.
- Stress management techniques.
- Social interaction such as day therapy.

Pharmacological

- Tricyclic antidepressants are usually contra-indicated as they are pro-arrhythmic.
- Most SSRIs seem to be helpful and safe, but recent data indicates that citalopram can prolong the Q-T interval which can increase the risk of fatal arrhythmia in people with HF.
- Trazodone (a serotonin antagonist and re-uptake inhibitor, SARI) and mirtazapine (a noradrenergic and specific serotonergic antidepressant, NaSSAs) appear to be safe in patients with HF.

Anxiety

Anxiety may be severe and persistent enough to become a chronic anxiety state, and may also be a presenting symptom of an anxiety-depression. Such patients may respond well to newer antidepressants with an anxiolytic action such as mirtazapine and avoid the risks of using benzodiazepines for all but acute anxiety episodes for short-term use.

- The more common situation in patients with HF is that they have realistic concerns about symptoms, increasing restrictions, and how they are going to cope.
- Anxiety can particularly exacerbate the symptom of breathlessness and superimposed panic attacks can be extremely distressing for patient and carer alike.
- Panic/breathlessness episodes can be a trigger for emergency, unwanted hospital admissions.
- It is important to recognize that patients may have specific anxieties which need to be explored.

ICDs and anxiety

Patients with ICDs in place may develop anxieties. For example, the uncertainty about whether it will discharge may prevent the patient going out and engaging in social activities, particularly if the device has previously discharged inappropriately. The threshold for discharge can be tailored for the individual; it may be appropriate to allow a delay to give time for loss of consciousness before a shock is delivered; however, there is a balance between maximizing effectiveness and minimizing fear of discharge. There may also be considerable anxieties around the time that switching off of the device becomes clinically recommended, as it is a sign of deteriorating disease. It is also important to remember that patients and their carers may have incorrect beliefs about the ability of the ICD to prevent death.

Management

- Active listening to patients' concerns; there may be specific anxieties that can be heard and resolved or signposted to specific agencies or relate to deeper issues.
- Anxiety/relaxation management including use of 'calming hand' techniques whereby the patient is encouraged to use their own hand as an immediate reminder of measures to calm panic (see Fig. 11.1).
- Pacing/prioritizing.
- Self-hypnosis, repeating a mantra.
- Complementary therapies such as massage or aromatherapy.
- Well-being interventions.
- Attention to dysfunctional breathing patterns.
- Judicious use of intermediate half-life benzodiazepines such as lorazepam or lormetazepam for panic episodes.
- Prepare a 'panic plan' for patients and carers to use, especially for OOH use.

Social problems

- Poor social support is associated with increased hospital admission and mortality.
- Single people with heart disease are more likely to be admitted and die earlier than those who are married.
- The same applies to married people who have a poor-quality relationship.

In a large interview study with HF patients, difficulties were encountered with a whole range of ADL:[4]

- Bathing, dressing.
- Shopping, cooking, and cleaning.
- Meaningful social interactions; holidays, hobbies, and visits to family and friends.
- Dealing with financial matters.
- Obtaining suitable housing and transport.

Financing paid help, if needed, can be hard. In the UK there is some non-means-tested state assistance in disability living or attendance allowances, but many patients find the process of application and appeal if turned down, daunting, unless they have an advocate. There is a 'fast track' route in the UK (DS1500), but this is often not claimed because of the uncertainties in prognosis.[5] This was complicated by the terminology on the DS1500 form appearing to refer solely to cancer, but this has now been rectified to include reference to advanced disease of other causes.

The choice to move to a nursing home can be deeply distressing for many, but so is struggling to maintain independence at home for the increasingly frail and isolated.

A key worker such as a HF nurse, community matron, or palliative care nurse can be invaluable in coordinating the multiprofessional team and crossing between health and social care settings to ensure a patient's needs are met. Such a role is particularly important when patients have little or no family support or live in deprived or rural areas.

The importance of informal carers in supporting patients with HF is often crucial and is highlighted in Chapter 15. Ensuring that these carers receive the necessary support to allow them to continue in their vital work can make the difference as to whether a patient stays in the community or is admitted to a health care facility. Thus it is important that as part of any overall assessment of patients with HF that the needs of the informal carer are also assessed.

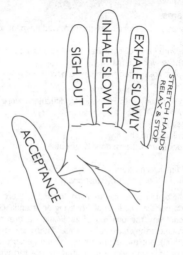

Fig. 11.1 Calming hand.

References

1 Buetow SA, Goodyear-Smith F, Coster GD (2001) Coping strategies in the self-management of chronic heart failure. *Family Practice* **18**, 117–22.
2 Guck TP, Elsasser GN, Kavan MG, Barone EJ (2003) Depression and congestive heart failure. *Congest Heart Fail* **9**, 163–9.
3 Gilbody S, Sheldon T, Wessely S (2006) Should we screen for depression? *BMJ* **332**, 1027–30.
4 Murray SA, Boyd K, Kendall M, Worth A, Benton TF, Clausen H (2002) Dying of lung cancer or cardiac failure: prospective qualitative interview study of patients and their carers in the community. *BMJ* **325**, 929.
5 Onac R, Fraser N, Johnson MJ (2010) State financial assistance for terminally ill patients—the discrepancy between cancer and heart failure. *Br J Cardiol* **17**, 73–5.

CPR and device therapy at the end of life

General issues

In the patient who is dying with end-stage cardiac disease, successful resuscitation from cardiopulmonary arrest is highly unlikely:
- The context is usually one of hepatorenal dysfunction, electrolyte disturbance, and myocardial depression.
- If cardiac output can be restored, the patient is highly unlikely to live to hospital discharge.
- If cardiac output can be restored there is a major risk of neurological damage, ranging from more subtle memory and processing cognitive problems through to gross neurological deficit.
- An ICD does not increase survival in patients with NYHA class IV HF, confirming this view. Many patients with NYHA IV HF do not die from a malignant arrhythmia but due to a slow progression of their HF.

In the dying patient, the decisions not to attempt CPR and to withdraw ICD support are analogous, and it is inconsistent to persist with one and not the other.

In the patient with better performance status, who is not in the dying phase:
- It may be appropriate to continue ICD support despite a DNACPR order, as there may be an acceptable outcome from immediate defibrillation, but any delay (such as would be inevitable from external CPR) would not be advisable.
- This should be discussed with the patient and the decision should be made having taken the risks and benefits into account.
- This should be reviewed regularly.

Patients with heart disease and their caregivers may have unrealistic expectations of what medical intervention can achieve at this stage, either from previous experience earlier on in the illness or from media portrayals of resuscitation.

CPR

There may also be uncertainty amongst patients, caregivers, and clinicians with regard to what treatments patients can request and what has to be discussed with a patient.

The joint statement from the BMA, Resuscitation Council (UK), and Royal College of Nursing (RCN) addresses these issues:[1]
- Clinicians are under no obligation to offer a futile intervention.
- Patients cannot demand a futile intervention.
- It is good practice to assess a patient's information needs and discuss management plans in the context of the patient's overall condition, including the caregivers with patient consent.
- If it is thought that it will cause unnecessary distress to the patient to discuss a DNACPR order, then the clinician is not obliged to do so.
- A discussion should never be avoided purely because this would cause discomfort for the clinician.
- Broad consent from the patient (if he or she has mental capacity to do so) to discuss management with their caregivers can be sought without explicitly itemizing the details of that management plan to the patient, if this is felt to be unnecessarily distressing and they do not wish to have this level of information.

Discussing DNACPR orders with patients
- A clinical decision based on benefits and burdens in the best interests of the patient should be taken by the clinical team.
- If it is deemed that an attempt at CPR is futile, then the discussion is *not* asking the patient whether they wish the clinical team to attempt CPR, i.e. the discussion is that the intervention is *not* being offered.
- Discussions should take place in the context of a more wide-reaching conversation about what can be offered to the patient at this stage of their illness rather than a bald 'taking away' of an option.
- Most are able to understand that only treatments which have a reasonable chance of benefiting the patient should be employed, rather than those that will not (such as cardiac surgery, further cardiac medication, insertion of devices, and an attempt at CPR).
- Decisions and conversations should be clearly documented in the patient's notes and communicated to other members of the team (including between primary and secondary care and ambulance services if the patient has requested to be discharged home to die).

Tailoring information to the individual patient
- It is important to assess the patient's information needs and how they are coping with their illness.
- Most patients value honesty if delivered with concern, although many clinicians worry about 'taking away hope' and find patient distress difficult.
- Moving a patient's goals from the hopelessly unrealistic to the hopefully achievable may *maintain* hope, and build trust with their clinician.
- Evidence from the fields of oncology and renal medicine shows that although these conversations are hard, on balance they are welcomed by patients and their caregivers.[2–4]

- Some, particularly elderly patients, may attach less importance to individual autonomy, and research has shown that some would not want an explicit acknowledgement of the imminence of death.[5]
- A proportion of patients cope with the situation by using denial.
- Complete denial is rare; usually discussion can be negotiated, preferably with the caregivers present.

Discussion with caregivers

- Ideally discussions can be held with the patient present; however, sometimes the patient is happy to discuss the situation openly, but the family isn't, or vice versa.
- Patient consent is required (if there is mental capacity), but broad permission to discuss the situation is all that is needed. Occasionally a patient may embargo specific issues from discussion, and this should be respected if it is non-negotiable.
- It may also be appropriate to discuss issues that are a concern for the family but the patient does not wish to be involved in the details—this may be particularly pertinent for those wishing to die at home, where, if a DNACPR is not made explicit to the caregivers, they may inappropriately call the emergency services.
- Caregivers may have unrealistic expectations of CPR and find it difficult that this will not be offered—sometimes using the terminology of 'allowing natural death' can help them understand that the patient is dying and the team will not be able to prevent this.
- Often the family are relieved that inappropriate and undignified interventions will not be attempted.

Withdrawal of ICD support

As people with HF reach an advanced stage in their illness a full assessment of the appropriateness of existing management, both pharmacological and device therapies, should take place.

Although the *majority* of patients imminently dying from HF do not die from tachyarrhythmias, if a patient develops a malignant tachyarrhythmia such as VT or VF on the background of end-stage HF it is unlikely that activation of an ICD will significantly prolong life, and there is a risk that there may be temporary restoration of cardiac output only for the ICD to discharge again. As such the patient's dying phase may be interrupted by multiple shocks from the ICD which are unpleasant for the patient, family, and staff.

Deactivation of the defibrillator needs to be considered where patients have either an internal defibrillator (ICD) or a CRTD. Pacemakers or CRT with a pacemaker only (i.e. CRTP) will not prolong life at this stage and will not cause the patient any discomfort. As such a pacemaker and a CRTP device can remain active.

This is often a difficult discussion to have with patients and their families even although the patient is approaching end of life care. Part of the difficulty is that this is often the first time deactivation of the defibrillator has been raised. Also patients and their families often have a relatively poor understanding of what a defibrillator is and how it works. Many patients feel that they will die immediately when their device is deactivated even although for the vast majority of patients this is not the case. The ideal scenario is that the defibrillator is deactivated and the ICD programmed to pacing mode only in a planned and controlled setting prior to any discharges occurring in the dying phase.

The Arrhythmia Alliance indications for deactivation are:[6]
• Continued use of an ICD is inconsistent with patient goals.
• Withdrawal of anti-arrhythmic medications.
• Imminent death (activation inappropriate in the dying phase).
• While an active DNACPR order is in force.[*]

As a general rule, if a patient is not for active resuscitation then their defibrillator in the majority of cases should be deactivated. What determines the difficulty of making the decision to deactivate a device is the patient's wishes and their VT burden. For those who have never or rarely used their device following implant then the decision to deactivate is much easier than for those with a high VT burden, as most will not tolerate VT and the device will no longer be active to provide therapy if needed.

---

[*] This is correct for the majority of patients but there may be specific circumstances where immediate defibrillation is likely to be of clinical benefit but any substantial delay for external CPR would be either futile or have a high risk of neurological compromise, for example a rural patient. This situation should be reviewed regularly, so the window of opportunity for the patient to be well enough to travel for deactivation is not missed.

The process of deactivation

The process of deactivation requires the following:

- Agreement by the usual care team in conjunction with cardiology that deactivation of the ICD is appropriate.
- Discussion with patient* and family emphasizing:
  - The device will no longer be able to provide life-saving therapy.
  - Turning off the device will not cause immediate death.
  - Turning off the device will not be painful, nor will its failure to function cause pain.
  - The ICD will continue to provide bradycardia support if needed but that this will not be painful and will not prolong life.
- A programmer compatible with the device.
- A header to be placed over the generator.
- Follow the programmer commands to deactivate the tachycardia therapies.

In the event of an emergency where the patient is experiencing recurrent shocks from their defibrillator and further shocks have been deemed inappropriate but formal device deactivation is not immediately possible then a strong magnet can be placed over the generator and this will deactivate most defibrillators (Box 12.1).

If magnet deactivation has been required the cardiology department should be contacted to arrange formal deactivation of the device. Local arrangements will be in place for OOH emergencies.

Box 12.1 Emergency defibrillator deactivation using a magnet

If a patient is dying with an active ICD and it starts to discharge:

- The ICD may be deactivated without disrupting pacemaker function by placing a magnet over the ICD.
- Tape a strong magnet over the generator box, usually located in the left or right subclavicular region. Do not remove the magnet from above the generator—it will only deactivate the generator whilst in position.
- It should be easily visible on examination.

The explanation to the patient and carer should be in the context of the overall stage of the disease and aim of care. The explanation should specifically state that turning off the ICD will not:

- Shorten life (unless the patient is in VT storm).
- Turn off the pacing function.
- Cause immediate death (unless the patient is in VT storm).
- Be painful.

Contact the cardiology department to arrange formal deactivation

---

* The decision to withdraw ICD support should always be discussed with the patient if they have mental capacity. If they do not, then the process outlined in the Mental Capacity Act 2005 (UK) should be followed. This is a non-invasive procedure and is a withdrawal of support and therefore written consent is *not* required; however, it is only appropriate that the patient understands what is going to happen and why.

Following device deactivation in either the controlled or emergency setting, anticipatory prescribing should be considered to avoid distress for the patient and carers in the event of further VT. Morphine and lorazepam are usually sufficient. In rare circumstances midazolam would be required.

Occasionally patients will insist that their device remains active and as long as they are deemed competent then this wish needs to be adhered to unless the clinical situation is such that medically it is felt not to be in the best interest of the patient. In most circumstances even if patients have requested that their device remain active there is most often an agreement regarding deactivation towards the very end of life.

Where patients are at home and wish to remain there, local protocols should be followed to allow for device deactivation to take place at home with the appropriate support network for the patient, family, and carers. A plan for end of life care should be in place with anticipatory prescribing to include the symptom management of further ventricular arrhythmias.

Following the death of a patient with any device (pacemaker, ICD, CRTP, or CRT-D) the mortuary/undertakers must be notified. For those patients where a cremation has been arranged the generator must be removed.

Points to consider

- Ideally, information should be given (either verbally or written) at the time of defibrillator insertion that there will come a time when the ICD will no longer provide appropriate benefit.
- Discussion should take place regarding deactivation, if the patient is willing, between the GP, cardiologist, and HFNS early in the palliation phase (Phase 2). Patients and their families need to become comfortable with the idea that appropriateness of the device remaining active will be continually reviewed.
- It is easier for deactivation to take place within the cardiology department so it is important that these discussions are planned at a time when the patient is still well enough to attend the hospital department.
- When this has not happened because deterioration has occurred quickly, or the patient has not allowed the conversation to take place, then local procedures need to be in place to facilitate reprogramming at the patient's bedside either in hospital, hospice, or at home.
- If the ICD is still active and there are no local procedures for immediate device deactivation at the patient's bedside, then access to magnetic deactivation should be made available.

Safety considerations with patients with ICDs

- It is safe to touch a patient even if their ICD is discharging.
- An ICD magnet is safe for clinicians and carers and should not affect bystanders with pacemakers as long as they don't lean close to the magnet.
- If a patient has died needing magnetic deactivation, do not remove the magnet until the ICD has been reprogrammed.
- Funeral directors will not be able to further prepare the body until the ICD has been permanently deactivated.

Further reading

British Heart Foundation discussion document on implantable cardioverter defibrillators in patients who are reaching the end of life. Available from the British Society for Heart Failure website (http://www.bsh.org.uk/portals/2/icd%20leaflet.pdf).

References

1 *Decisions relating to cardiopulmonary resuscitation: a joint statement from the British Medical Association, the Resuscitation Council (UK) and the Royal College of Nursing.* British Medical Association, BMA House, Tavistock Square, London WC1H 9JP, UK (1 October 2007).
2 Davison SN, Simpson C (2006) Hope and advance care planning in patients with end stage renal disease: qualitative interview study. *BMJ* **333**, 886.
3 Fallowfield LJ, Jenkins VA, Beveridge HA (2002) Truth may hurt but deceit hurts more: communication in palliative care. *Palliat Med* **16**, 297–303.
4 Michel DM, Moss AH (2005) Communicating prognosis in the dialysis consent process: a patient-centered, guideline-supported approach. *Adv Chronic Kidney Dis* **12**, 196–201.
5 Gott M, Small N, Barnes S, Payne S, Seamark D (2008) Older people's views of a good death in heart failure: implications for palliative care provision. *Soc Sci Med* **67**, 1113–21.
6 Arrhythmia Alliance *Implantable cardioverter defibrillators (ICDs) in dying patients.* (http://www.hruk.org.uk/Docs/ICD%20Deactivation%20Leaflet-Arrhythmia%20Alliance.pdf).

Chapter 13

Care of the dying

General issues

- The process of recognizing dying follows the principle of assessing a patient's current presentation within the context of their individual illness trajectory as discussed in 📖 Chapter 3.
- There may be uncertainty, but this need not preclude the patient receiving excellent symptom care and being gently involved in honest discussions regarding the gravity of the situation.
- If there is continued active treatment, this should be reviewed daily by a member of the usual medical team able to make decisions regarding treatment withdrawal, as failure to respond is one of the signs of the dying phase.
- An end of life care tool, the LCP or local equivalent, is a prompt for care and a clinical decision aid. The LCP was developed initially for the hospital setting but is now adapted for use in the community, nursing home, and hospice.[1]
- The LCP has the facility for trials of active therapy to be given, provided there are clear rationales given, goals indicated, and timescales set—such trials are documented as a 'variance'. This should allow clinical discretion and acknowledge the inherent clinical uncertainty, but minimizes the risk of ambivalent and inappropriate prescribing in a dying patient simply because clinicians have not allowed themselves to recognize that the patient is likely to be dying.
- The five main symptoms (breathlessness, agitation, respiratory tract secretions, nausea, and pain) appear to be in common with patients dying from cancer and the prompts of care used in the LCP seem to be applicable to people dying from HF.[2]

General approach to care of the dying

Initial assessment

- Full assessment of the extent of disease, symptoms, and, where possible, understanding of illness/levels of distress is key. This will often help target specific symptom measures, e.g. oxygen for hypoxic confusion, or catheterization for urinary retention-induced agitation. Inappropriate oral medication should be discontinued, and prn medication for symptom measures written up on the drug chart and prescribed to be administered SC (Table 13.1).
- Full assessment of the family's understanding of the stage of illness, what treatment is being employed and why—and which treatments are not and why not. Often there is poor understanding and great overestimation of what can be realistically offered. There is also little understanding of signs of impending death, and time spent at this stage is often needed. The family may also be grateful for practical information such as where to get a shower, or food and drink, or a bed for the night. There may be specific family or patient religious or spiritual requirements at this time of which the clinical team need to be aware.
- The LCP contains a prompt to check that an ICD, if present, has been reprogrammed to pacemaker mode only, or deactivated completely if there is no bradycardia indication. A useful booklet from the British Heart Foundation (BHF) with information regarding ICDs and the end of life is available for health care professionals.[3] However, the only patient and carer ICD information available (from the Arrhythmia Alliance) does not contain any information about end of life or the need for reprogramming.[4]
- A DNACPR decision should be documented. This is particularly important if the patient has expressed a wish to die at home. If this is the case, then this should be clearly discussed with the patient's GP before transfer home and local arrangements put in place to prevent OOH emergency ambulance services attempting CPR in the event of death at home.

Ongoing assessment

- The five key symptoms and any others noted at initial assessment will be reviewed every 6hr and addressed if the patient is not settled. In addition, bladder and bowel comfort are checked twice daily. Skin and mouth care are also reviewed.
- Psychological state and understanding of family, and patient if appropriate, is reviewed regularly. Ongoing care regarding this aspect is important—often other family members that were not involved in the initial discussions 'appear' at this stage, or family disharmony about goals of care or understanding about the stage of the illness can become apparent. Time spent in explanation and listening to grief can prevent problems in bereavement, and complaints arising out of misunderstandings about care.
- The patient should have a medical review daily and therefore if the patient's condition should improve, there is the option to take them off the LCP if this is deemed appropriate.

- If the patient is needing more than two prn doses of a medication in 24hr, then consider a continuous SC infusion by syringe driver (Table 13.2).

Table 13.1 Anticipatory prescribing for prn medication

Symptom	Drug (SC stat dose as needed)
Pain	Diamorphine 2.5mg
Breathlessness	Midazolam 2.5–5mg (use first line, unless apnoeic spells are a cause of distress to the patient, in which case try diamorphine first)
	Diamorphine 2.5mg (if apnoeic spells are distressing)
	Furosemide* (the patient should always be examined for signs of pulmonary oedema and, unless anuric, a parenteral dose of loop diuretic given and repeated as necessary after 2hr)
Agitation	Midazolam 2.5–5mg
Nausea/vomiting	Haloperidol 1.5mg
Excess respiratory secretions	Hyoscine butylbromide 20mg (although anticholinergic drugs should be avoided in HF, in the last few days/hours of life, symptom benefit should take precedence and is highly unlikely to materially affect survival)

*Dose as indicated by the individual situation.

Table 13.2 Suggested medication for continuous infusion

Symptom	Drug (suggested starting doses—to be titrated to effect using additional stat doses if needed to achieve comfort)
Pain	5–10mg diamorphine/24hr via syringe driver, or 0.5–1mg alfentanil/24hr if renal dysfunction
Breathlessness	10mg midazolam/24hr via syringe driver. If the patient requires more than two doses of parenteral diuretic for pulmonary oedema then an infusion should be set up. For IV infusion, 10mg/hr should be started. For a SC infusion, then use the 24hr oral or IV dose and infuse over 24hr
Agitation	10mg midazolam/24hr via syringe driver
Nausea/vomiting	1.5–3mg haloperidol/24hr via syringe driver
Excess respiratory secretions	60mg hyoscine butylbromide/24hr via syringe driver

SC administration of furosemide

Patients with advanced HF often need parenteral administration of loop diuretic when the gut becomes too oedematous to efficiently absorb the medication. There is some evidence that a continuous infusion of loop diuretic is more effective and better tolerated than daily bolus injections.

For those at the very end of life, however, it is difficult to provide a home IV service as many areas do not have community staff trained to give IV injections. It is even more difficult to provide a home continuous IV infusion service; although there are indwelling IV catheters they carry significant risks and costs. Even for straightforward bolus injections, many patients at the end of life find the IV route uncomfortable, or even lose this route completely as they become more unwell.

Therefore, recently, attention has been given to the possibility of using the SC route for administering furosemide in selected patients with advanced HF:

- Normal volunteers randomized to receive bolus SC injections of normal saline or furosemide showed an increased diuresis and natriuresis with furosemide compared with saline.[5]
- A case series of decompensated patients with HF demonstrated diuresis and natriuresis following SC administration of furosemide.[6]
- A case series of patients with advanced HF demonstrated weight loss, prevention of hospital admission from community or hospice, and use in the dying patient.[7]

Further experience and research are needed to confirm the role of this route of administration, but given that the infrastructure is in place for this to be rolled out across the NHS (every community nurse already has training and access with regard to the portable pumps required for continuous SC infusion), this could be a useful way of supporting patients with advanced HF in their preferred place of care and easing the morbidity associated with IV use. In addition, many hospices are more at ease with continuous SC infusion than IV infusion. Thus hospice admission for HF patients towards the end of life requiring parenteral diuretics may be more of an option if SC infusion was a possibility.

Care after death

- Prompts for care can be tailored to local protocol and include procedures for handing over personal property, giving and explaining death certificates, requirements for registration of death, as well as giving information and literature about death and bereavement.
- The LCP provides a clearly identifiable place in the clinical record to document verification and confirmation of death with record of who signed the certificate and cremation forms if relevant.
- Removal of devices (see 📖 Chapter 12) should be clearly documented, and knowledge of local policies is important.
- Patients with HF often have much comorbidity and making sure that all clinicians who were involved in their care are informed of their death is important—a clinic appointment arriving in the home of the deceased a few months later can be distressing for the bereaved.

Case history

Mrs H was an 82-year-old lady who had had a significant MI 8 years previously complicated by a VF cardiac arrest in the ambulance as she was taken to hospital. After a stormy inpatient stay her condition stabilized and she was discharged. Over the next few months she improved and was able to manage at home and tolerated optimal cardiac medical treatment.

However, a year ago, her ACE inhibitor and beta-blocker had to be repeatedly down-titrated because of symptomatic hypotension and since a further MI 3 months ago she has not managed any, and has struggled to maintain her independence at home.

After discussion between Mrs H, her GP, and her cardiologist, the palliative physician was asked to see her in her flat because she had become very breathless on minimal exertion, severely fatigued, and oedematous despite escalating doses of oral loop diuretic and the addition of a thiazide. She now has significant renal dysfunction. Despite comprehensive home support with carers three times a day and night, with 'meals on wheels', a cleaner, and a gardener, she doubted that she would be able to continue living at home. She expressed a wish for no further hospital treatment and was aware that she was 'near the end'. She agreed to come into the local hospice for a trial of parenteral loop diuretic although she understood that this is unlikely to be successful. She agreed that an attempt at CPR should not be made. She contacted her son in South Africa who arranged to fly to the UK the following day. She has also contacted her church minister who is a strong source of support.

Over the next 48hr, she became more hypotensive with poor perfusion. She became bedbound, profoundly fatigued, sleeping most of the time. Her fluid overload worsened despite continuous infusion of furosemide. Her breathlessness started to make her agitated and distressed. She needed 2 stat doses of 2.5mg midazolam to settle her and a syringe driver of 10mg midazolam/24hr was commenced. As she also had some discomfort from pressure sores 0.5mg alfentanil/24hr was added. The continuous infusion of furosemide was withdrawn at this stage.

She was passing very little urine and had expressed a wish to avoid a catheter if possible. She was therefore nursed with a barrier cream and pads. She was turned only to avoid further marking of her skin, and regular use of emollients continued to prevent further breakdown. Her mouth was kept clean by using sponges moistened with water.

She died peacefully 5 days after admission to the hospice with her son and his wife at her side.

References

1 *Liverpool Care Pathway for the dying patient.* Marie Curie Palliative Care Institute, Liverpool (http://www.liv.ac.uk/mcpcil/liverpool-care-pathway/)

2 Marie Curie Palliative Care Institute Liverpool (MCPCIL) in collaboration with the Clinical Standards Department of the Royal College of Physicians (RCP) (2009) *National care of the dying audit—hospitals (NCDAH). Round 2. 2008-9.* 1-91. Supported by the Marie Curie Cancer Care and the Department of Health End of Life Care Programme (http://www.liv.ac.uk/mcpcil/liverpool-care-pathway/national-care-of-dying-audit.htm)

3 Beattie JM (2007) *Implantable cardioverter defibrillators in patients who are reaching the end of life.* British Heart Foundation, London (download from http://publications.bhf.org.uk/publications/view-publication.aspx?ps=1000155)

4 Arrhythmia Alliance *Implantable cardioverter defibrillators (ICDs) in dying patients.* (http://www.hruk.org.uk/Docs/ICD%20Deactivation%20Leaflet-Arrhythmia%20Alliance.pdf).

5 Verma AK, da Silva JH, Kuhl DR (2004) Diuretic effects of subcutaneous furosemide in human volunteers: a randomized pilot study. *Ann Pharmacother* **38**, 544–9.

6 Goenaga MA, Millet M, Sanchez E, Garde C, Carrera JA, Arzellus E (2004) Subcutaneous furosemide. *Ann Pharmacother* **38**, 1751.

7 Zacharias H, Raw J, Nunn A, Parsons S, Johnson MJ (2011) Is there a role for subcutaneous furosemide in the community and hospice management of end-stage heart failure? *Palliat Med* **25**, 658–63.

Spiritual and religious care

Introduction

- The care of any patient, and specifically of one who is approaching death, must encompass the physical, psychological, social, and spiritual aspects of that person.
- Spirituality is about making sense of what is happening to someone. It has to do with an individual's sense of peace and connection to others and their belief about the meaning of life. It is likely to be heightened at times of crisis such as facing a life-limiting illness or in the face of certain death.
- Spirituality may be found through an organized religion or in other ways.
- Religion is defined as a specific set of beliefs and practices, usually within an organized group. It may include ritual of worship or expression of faith, which varies with different beliefs and which helps that individual express their spirituality. It is important to differentiate the two, as a person who has no religious belief or needs may welcome spiritual care that affirms their humanity and supports their exploration of meaning, while not wishing any religious ritual.
- It is helpful to know if the patient has any spiritual or religious beliefs or practices, and how much of a source of strength they are to that individual and therefore how they might help him or her during their remaining life. It is not uncommon for transient loss of faith at this time and patients should be asked if they wish to see a chaplain or religious leader.
- End of life issues can challenge a patient's beliefs or religious values resulting in high levels of spiritual distress. Some believe their illness is a punishment for some previous misdemeanour, which may result in increased distress and loss of faith.

Spiritual care

Spiritual care is not just the facilitation of an appropriate ritual but engaging with an individual's search for existential meaning, as reflected in the existential domain of the McGill Quality of Life Questionnaire.[1]

Spiritual care is embedded within the holistic care of patient, family, and professional staff that palliative care embraces, yet it is often omitted or only has lip service paid to it. This may be through ignorance, embarrassment, lack of confidence, or fear of opening a conversation that the individual has neither the time nor the personal resources to deal with.

This is worrying and unnecessary, as all members of the multidisciplinary cardiac team who care for the dying patient can reach out to their patients' spiritual needs through normal practice and contact with patients. Often patients' spiritual needs are expressed at a time when pastoral or chaplaincy staff are not present. Frequently, this will be when people are at their most vulnerable, such as while being washed or having dressings changed, yet individuals will trust the staff member sufficiently to express their deep concerns—maybe with a question relating to their death.

Such opportunities are precious and should be responded to. This may involve holding on to the silence, or listening and enabling the patient to continue their questioning or tell their story, or through touch and an honest meeting of the eyes. For the patient it is the professional 'staying with them' at a time of need or distress that counts. It is also possible to offer further spiritual support from chaplaincy staff if the patient wishes, but it is equally important not to miss the opportunity in everyday practice.

Spirituality and spiritual distress

- Spirituality relates to the way people make sense of the world around them.
- It is about finding meaning in life.
- The knowledge or fear of the closeness of death is likely to bring those aspects of our being sharply into focus.
- Everyone has a spiritual dimension, though not all have spiritual needs.
- If spiritual distress is not recognized and attended to, it may lead to difficult symptom control, particularly pain control.
- Spiritual distress may express itself as terminal agitation or difficult and unrelieved pain.
- Relief of spiritual distress may be crucial to the 'healing' of an individual as they approach their death, and such healing will enhance their quality of life and aid symptom control.

Religious care

Religious care enables the person to express their spirituality through appropriate ritual and religious practice.

Assessing spiritual and religious needs

- Assessment of spiritual needs ideally should take place prior to the dying phase as patients are unlikely to have the energy to address such issues and maintain concentration as death draws closer.
- Open questions such as 'how do you deal or cope with life when faced with tough and difficult situations?' or 'is there anything that gives you a particular sense of meaning to your life?' or 'are you at peace?'[2] let the patient know you are willing to engage in a discussion about spiritual matters and can be used to open a discussion.
- It is also important to gauge how important this is in the person's life, so you might ask 'how important is this (or your faith) in your life?'.
- If the person tells you of their faith this gives you the opportunity to ask if they would like to see a 'faith leader' and if so to ensure the chaplaincy team is aware of this.
- They should also be asked how they would like these matters to be dealt with in their health care or could be asked 'are there any particular religious customs I need to know about to help you?'.

Giving spiritual support includes:
- Being led by the patient.
- Listening actively.
- Using silence.
- Avoiding judgement.
- Liaison with appropriate pastoral support or religious leaders.

Spiritual and religious well-being is associated with quality of life, with some research showing that these beliefs can promote a more positive mental attitude that can enhance a patient's remaining quality of life by:
- Reducing anxiety.
- Reducing depression.
- Reducing a sense of isolation and 'aloneness'.
- Facilitating better acceptance and adjustment to their illness.

Spiritual distress may contribute to the patient's inability to cope with end of life issues. Knowing the role that religion and spirituality play in the patient's life may help caregivers understand the beliefs that affect the patient's responses to end of life issues.

A practical summary
- Try to ensure privacy and sufficient time.
- Ask what is important in the person's life or if anything gives their life meaning.
- Find out how important this is to them.
- If a patient tells you of their faith, ask what kind of support they would like.
- Discover what if any religious practices are important for their spiritual well-being, e.g. the opportunity to pray in a particular way.
- Find out if there are particular things to be avoided or others that are important in their faith life.
- Find out if they have a minister of religion whom they would like contacted at any time.

- At an appropriate time ascertain whether they have an up to date will and, if not, if they wish to produce one.
- Be prepared to discuss their funeral wishes if they would like.
- When the time is right enquire about practice around death itself and afterwards—this will depend on the person's response to previous questions.

Possible spiritual issues for the patient with end-stage cardiac disease

What's in a name?

The term 'heart failure' can be very emotive; the term 'heart' is central to our sense of self, our seat of emotion, our being, and life itself. Also the word 'failure' in lay language is laden with meaning; we 'fail' an examination or a marriage. Whilst it is not suggested that the term is avoided, the clinician needs to be aware of this when discussing the condition with the patient and family. In addition, patients with HF have often had previously poor communication with health care professionals (see 📖 Chapter 4) and have a consequently poor understanding of their condition that feeds into a possible perception that 'the very heart of me has failed'.

A source of unmet need

Qualitative research[3–5] has shown spiritual issues in people with heart disease to be:

- A source of unmet need.
- Important.
- Inextricably linked to many other problems.

Long experience of living with chronic illness and disability has led to:

- Hopelessness.
- Loss of purpose.
- Isolation.
- Altered self-image.

These were general to most people living with HF whereas religious concerns were apparent in only a few.

As the illness progresses and the reality of death becomes closer, then the search for meaning in life can become deeper, including a need for forgiveness. This can be a lonely struggle for patients, sometimes over months, unshared with health professionals or even immediate family.

Sources of strength

However, despite the difficulties, studies demonstrate impressive resilience and the ability to find strength from a variety of sources:

- Family and other relationships.
- Those who were religious, from church support and their personal faith.

Cultural issues and spiritual support

In every culture loss is accompanied by grief, although it may be expressed in a variety of ways. In a multicultural society patients have different attitudes towards discussing death. No individual can be separated from the context in which they live, be it family, medical, or wider social contexts. It can be a frightening and bewildering experience for those who do not speak the same language as those who care for them, and patients can be left feeling very isolated and misunderstood.

The cultural and religious backgrounds of patients may play an integral role in their interpretation of death and the coping mechanisms they use.

Many view death as a transition rather than extinction so it can be seen that religion and spirituality can influence one's concept of death and dying by offering a reason for being and a framework in which to interpret the inevitable.

Communication

Effective communication is needed when working in a cross-cultural setting. Otherwise one cannot check that a patient has fully understood the implications of end of life care discussions.

We need to recognize the following:

- Mourning behaviour and rituals must be understood within the bereaved individual's religious and cultural background.
- Having prior knowledge of cultural issues, including how the patient's cultural, spiritual, or religious beliefs influence the way they think about caring for the dying, avoids burdening the patient or the family with the additional role of being educators.
- We may not know how patients maintain good health, what they believe to be the cause of their illness, and whether religion or spiritual beliefs play a role in their illness, but we can establish this by admitting we are unfamiliar with their culture and asking how best we can help them.
- If language barriers are hampering good communication, the services of an independent interpreter should be sought.

People expect their cultural values and way of life to be respected and understood, which is why we should try to think in terms of similarities between cultures rather than differences.

Religious practices of different faiths in relation to end of life care

Table 14.1 gives a summary of the end of life practices of different faiths.

It is not possible to cover all shades of each religion in this short section, it is important always to ask the individual and family what their personal practice and religious needs are, and not to assume that they will conform to a 'norm' as described here or in other texts.

Buddhism

There are a number of different schools of Buddhism, any of which may be represented among HF patients and all of whom practise meditation. Buddhism teaches the inevitability of death. Therefore, a practitioner is likely to be calm and dignified as they face death. Though relief of pain is acceptable, analgesics and sedatives may be declined towards the end of life, and sometimes earlier, so as to die with a clear mind.

Euthanasia is rejected, but withdrawal of medical intervention when death is near is not seen as immoral, so withdrawing ICD support, for example, should not normally raise a religious problem for a Buddhist.

Customs at end of life include:
- Inviting a Buddhist teacher or monk to be present with the patient.
- Peace and quiet for meditation to ensure a calm state of mind as dying.
- Single-sex room, particularly for monks.
- Listening to Buddhist chants as death approaches.

Christianity

Within Christianity there are also a number of denominations with different traditions. Central to Christianity is the belief that Jesus Christ was the son of God and that he rose from the dead following crucifixion. Christians believe in life after death. Attitudes to death will vary from a rejoicing acceptance to great distress, and all shades between; distress may be associated with feelings of guilt concerning unforgiven sins or a loss of faith. Many (but not all) are helped by seeing a priest or minister of their own or similar denomination for prayer, which may be accompanied by confession, absolution, holy communion, or anointing. It can be important for a Roman Catholic to receive the sacrament of the sick from a Roman Catholic priest.

Analgesia and sedation can be accepted for relief of pain and suffering but some Christians may wish to remain clear in their thinking and decline medication, or delay its use to give time for repentance or reconciliation. Intentionally bringing about death is forbidden; but attempts to prolong life at all costs are not commensurate with Christian beliefs either.

Customs at end of life include:
- The sacrament of confession with absolution.
- Receiving communion.
- Laying on of hands.
- Anointing with oil.
- Prayer with patient and family.

Hinduism

Hinduism is a family of beliefs embracing a very wide diversity of traditions but with common beliefs relating to transition to another life either with reincarnation, life in heaven with God, or absorption into Brahman:

A good death is an important part of spiritual life. Religious life plays a significant part in physical life and in this context suffering can be seen as a reflection of wrongs committed.

Purification of the body is very important, particularly to bathe in running water, as part of a daily routine. Many will wish to do so before praying in the morning. Most Hindus will wish to have physical care carried out by carers of the same sex as themselves and it is important that this is respected.

A good death occurs peacefully in old age, having put affairs in order, said goodbye, and resolved conflict. The 'old age' aspect of a good death can cause problems for younger Hindus who are dying.

Some Hindus will stop eating and drinking as they approach death to purify the body and spirit. Analgesia and sedation may also be declined to keep the mind clear as they prepare for death. Euthanasia is not permitted.

Customs at end of life include:
- Placing the mattress on the floor at end of life.
- Preference for death at home.
- Having family present while dying.
- Reading from Hindu holy books and hymns.
- Being given Ganges water and a Tulsi leaf in the mouth at the time of death.
- Family likely to want to wash the body after death.

Islam

Followers of Islam, known as Muslims, believe in one God and the presence of prophets to guide the faithful, the last and most influential of whom was Muhammad. They see the historic record of his actions and teachings as tools for interpreting the Qur'an. Muslims also believe in a final day of judgement. 'Islam' means submitting to the will of God. Most Muslims are strict about abiding by Islamic law with respect to diet, prayer, fasting, etc. Modesty is important in nursing care, with a preference for same-sex carers. Prayer is said five times a day, facing Mecca and after washing with running water. These aspects of religious life will be important at the end of life and professional carers must ask the patient what their wishes are.

Fasting during Ramadan from dawn to dusk is incumbent on Muslims in health. Many who are terminally ill may choose to fast a certain amount, particularly as it is also a time for resolving disputes. Meals will need to be provided before dawn and after dusk. As fasting includes taking anything into the body, medication may also be declined during the hours of daylight.

Muslims believe in life after death, that suffering is part of God's plan, and accept death as His will. For the individual, as in other religions, this can be a great comfort but also for some a source of guilt and distress.

Euthanasia is prohibited, but pain relief can be given and futile treatment withdrawn.

However, suffering may be considered important to endure with regard to entering Paradise after death. Analgesia and sedation may be declined to keep the mind clear during preparation for death.

Customs at end of life include:

- Wish to die facing Mecca (south-east in UK).
- Family or other Muslims to recite prayers.
- After death the body only to be touched by Muslims.
- If staff have to touch the body it should be while wearing disposable gloves.
- The person's face should be placed towards the right shoulder.

Sikhism

Sikhs believe in one omnipresent and infinite God. They see death as a natural process and part of the cycle of life, progressing on the path to unity with God through successive reincarnations. The 'five ks'—kesh, long hair; kacchera, shorts; kanga, small wooden comb; kara, bracelet; kirpan, sword—must be worn by baptised Sikhs. Many will be vegetarian, although others only decline pork and beef.

As a Sikh is dying, relatives and friends may wish to recite from their holy book. When death occurs, they should recite the name of God. Sikhs believe that the soul moves on to meet the supreme soul, God. Overt expression of grief is discouraged.

Cremation is preferred as the body is only considered to be an empty shell, but if this is not possible, burial at sea is acceptable; that is a defined place for burial and a gravestone are discouraged; ashes are disposed of in the nearest river. Before cremation, the body is washed with yoghurt and water, dressed in clean clothes and with the Five Ks, whilst those present recite from the holy book. The body is then transferred to the coffin.

Euthanasia is not allowed but withdrawal of futile treatment is.

Customs at the end of life include:

- Death is seen as a time for praising God in accordance with the teachings of code of conduct, the Rahit Maryada. After someone dies, if the body is on a bed it should not be moved and no light should be placed next to it.
- The family read the Holy Book continuously for 48hr or in stages which must be completed within 1 week and end on the day of the funeral.
- Hymns are sung in preparation for the cremation of the body.

Judaism

The attitude of Jews to death and dying is based on convictions. They believe the body belongs to God and that therefore there is an obligation to try to heal it. Most Jews will want to know the truth about their illness so they can plan well. Jewish law is binding and Jews may wish to consult family or rabbi before making serious treatment decisions.

Suicide and therefore euthanasia are against Jewish law. It is, however, generally permissible to withdraw life-sustaining treatment in the presence of a terminal illness, if in the patient's best interest. Pain control is permissible as long as not given with the intent of shortening life, though patients may prefer to maintain clarity of thought and decline analgesia.

Customs at end of life include the following:
- Attention to the bereaved may be greater than that to dying person.
- A request to see a rabbi is an individual decision and not necessary for ritual.
- Prayers may be said.
- Traditionally, closing the eyes, laying the arms straight, and binding up the lower jaw are done by a family member.
- After death the body is placed on the floor, feet towards the door, covered with a white sheet, and a candle lit.
- The body cannot be moved on the Sabbath (Saturday) so it is important to have anticipated this.
- Watchers stay with the body until burial.

Summary

This has been a brief sketch of selected features of some faiths. Reference to more extensive texts and to the relevant faith community leaders may be necessary to ensure optimal religious care. All hospitals and hospices have access to chaplaincy or pastoral support teams; these will be an important source of information to local teams and should be used.
- The care of the individual is unique and assumptions based on religious faith should not be made.
- Patients and families should be asked their needs and preferences.
- Care teams should endeavour to honour those wishes.

Cultural resource and further reading

Lancet Viewpoint Series: End of life issues for different religions (2005) *Lancet* **366**, 682–6, 774–9, 862–5, 952–5, 1045–8, 1132–5, 1235–7.

References

1 Speck P, Higginson IJ, Addington-Hall JM (2004) Spiritual needs in health care. *BMJ* **329**, 123–4.
2 Steinhauser KE, Voils CI, Glipp EC et al. (2006) 'Are you at peace?': one item to probe spiritual concerns at the end of life. *Arch Intern Med* **166**, 101–5.
3 Murray SA, Boyd K, Kendall M et al. (2002) Dying of lung cancer or cardiac failure: prospective qualitative interview study of patients and their carers in the community. *BMJ* **325**, 929–32.
4 Fitchett G, Murphy PE, Kim J et al. (2004) Religious struggle: prevalence, correlates and mental health risks in diabetic, congestive heart failure, and oncology patients. *Int J Psychiatry Med* **34**, 179–96.
5 Murray SA, Kendall M, Boyd K et al. (2004) Exploring the spiritual needs of people dying of lung cancer or heart failure: a prospective qualitative interview study of patients and their carers. *Palliat Med* **18**, 39–45.

Table 14.1 End of life customs of the different religions*

Religion	Diet	Particular	Customs around dying	Actions after death	Method of disposal	Autopsy
Buddhism	Many vegetarian	Peace & quiet to allow meditation	Wish to be calm & fully conscious: may request monk to chant	Contact priest immediately; body should not be removed till he arrives	Burial or cremation	May be permitted if religious teacher allows
Christianity	Individual; no forbidden foods	None	May wish to receive absolution, holy communion, or anointing from priest or minister	No special requirements	Burial or cremation	Permitted; with respect to body
Hindu	Strict handling rules; no beef	May prefer mattress on floor; home death preferred	May call Hindu priest for holy rites; Ganges water and Tulsi leaf placed in mouth	Family to wash (if done by health care workers, must wear gloves); jewellery left with body	Cremation as soon as possible	Is permitted
Islam	Special preparation; vegetarian or 'halal' meat; no pork	Modesty & cleanliness very important. Washing in running water before prayer. Fully dressed at night	If possible to sit or lie facing Mecca; privacy for continued daily prayer; declaration of faith made	Body washed by same sex Muslim; non-Muslims need permission to touch body; body kept covered in clean white cotton garments	Burial only, within 24h	Permitted if required by law

Judaism	Orthodox kosher meals; check individual requirements	Dying person should not be left alone	Those present may recite psalms; rabbi not essential but may be called	Cover body with white sheet; body laid on floor, feet to the door, candle by head	Burial usually as soon as possible	Only if required by law. Minimally invasive; return of organs to body
Sikhism	Usually decline beef & pork; many vegetarian	May like to recite or listen to hymns from sikh hly book	Should die with God's name being recited	Do not trim hair or beard; cover body with plain white cloth; leave 5 Ks† with body; family members to wash body	Cremation as soon as possible	Permitted if required by law

* The six faith communities described all prohibit euthanasia but allow the withdrawal of futile treatment. Pain relief is also allowed by all, though practitioners may choose to decline it or sedation so as to maintain as clear a mind as possible, and there may be different interpretations of what is allowed by different practitioners.

† Five Ks: kesh, long hair: kacchera, shorts: kanga, small wooden comb: kara, bracelet: kirpan, sword.

From Brown E, Chambers J, Eggeling C (2007) *End of life care in nephrology: from advanced disease to bereavement.* Oxford University Press, Oxford. Reproduced with permission of Oxford University Press.

Supporting carers

The role of carers

While clinical care is supervised by health professionals, the largest proportion of everyday care in the UK is provided by informal carers. More than 5 million people offer some form of care, substituting for a professional service that would cost more than £70 billion annually.[1] These are usually family members, particularly spouses or children, but also include family friends or neighbours.

Carers UK has defined carers as people who 'provide unpaid care by looking after an ill, frail or disabled family member, friend or partner' (http://www.carersuk.org/).

Impact of chronic HF on patients

- Chronic HF often confers escalating care needs on the affected individual as the condition evolves and symptoms worsen as the patient declines towards death.
- Chronic HF is often associated with multiple refractory symptoms linked to several comorbidities creating increased dependency despite complex therapy.[2,3]
- Patients with chronic HF are often elderly and can become increasingly reliant on their spouses, who may also be elderly, or other family members to assist them in undertaking ADL such as washing and dressing, as well as maintaining nutrition and hydration.

Impact of chronic HF on carers

In their medical support role informal carers often are required to monitor fluid balance and supervise the administration of complex medication regimes, transport the patient to and from hospital appointments, and to decide when to call for help in the face of apparent clinical deterioration.

Beyond these physical and organizational roles, often regarded as a family duty, the caregiver burden can be compounded by:

• Understandable anxiety about the declining health of their loved one.
• Feelings of isolation if their usual social networks are disrupted.
• Economic disadvantage if work activity has to be limited by caring responsibilities.

If the principal carer has been the major breadwinner in the household and this function is now denied, there may be financial implications for the whole family. HF patients can become sensitive to their dependency and often have concerns about the effects their illness is imposing on their family carers.[4]

It is recognized that adopting a caring role brings with it risks of physical or psychological morbidity and higher mortality.[5]

Elements of carer burden and risk

As gauged by the Caregiver Reactions Assessment Scale,[6] the major domains of the carer burden in HF are perceived as:

- Disturbed daily schedule.
- Loss of physical strength.
- Lack of family support.

Characteristics of those at particular risk include:

- Older age.
- Symptoms of depression.
- Pre-existing medical conditions.
- Declining physical well-being.
- Caring for other relatives.
- Caring for someone with multiple comorbidities.
- Feeling abandoned or unsupported.
- Contributing excessive hours.

In 2001, two-thirds of all carers were caring > 20hr/week and one-fifth cared for > 50 hr/week.[1] Identification of these subsets and the provision of enhanced professional care and respite may reduce carer burdens.

Studies of evolving household and family structures suggest that the pool of carers will contract and underscore the need for prospective professional care planning to accommodate an increasingly aged and clinically complex population.[7]

Supporting informal carers

Carers need access to a whole range of services to allow them to continue and extend their role and the vital work that they do for society at large.

Integration of social care with health care is central to cohesive management of the overall care needs of individual patients with HF. However, coordination of care between agencies is often difficult despite the widespread realization that, for example, provision of timely benefit entitlements or prompt access to equipment can have a major impact in allowing carers to keep patients out of acute care facilities. All carers have a right to assessment by a social worker but the provision of such statutory services is patchy at best.

Carer support is enshrined in the White Paper 'Developing a national care service',[8] and commissioning tools for social care are also available but have not yet generated the joined up approach to supporting carers that will be required to maximize the benefit that carers can provide to patients and to the health care service.

A successful model for providing social care support to the carers of patients with end-stage HF has been developed in the Care-Plus Project, sponsored by the King's Fund, in the London Borough of Tower Hamlets (http://www.carerscentretowerhamlets.org.uk/). A dedicated project coordinator provides bespoke carer support acting as a link to service providers and facilitating fast-track access to health and social care services. The evaluation report on the Care-Plus Project has been submitted to the National Institute for Health and Clinical Excellence (NICE) for consideration as a replicable model of service delivery.

Disease-related variability

While the specific characteristics of the patient, carer, and their social context affect the carer burden, this also changes dynamically in parallel with the stage of the illness and the patient's unique disease trajectory. Patterns of clinical deterioration are highly variable, making it very challenging to conduct forward planning for end of life care for individual patients using existing planning models, many of which have evolved out of more predictable cancer trajectories.[9] Goodlin has proposed a different representation of a disease trajectory that reflects current comprehensive HF care, and which may prove more suitable in the future to frame carer information and support (see 📖 Chapter 3).[10]

Disease trajectory (Fig. 15.1)

Phase 1

- Symptom onset, diagnosis, and initiation of medical treatment.
- This may be linked to an emergency admission with HF as a new diagnosis. Some patients may die at this point.

Carer needs

During this phase, both patients and carers need education on the nature of HF, the treatment options, dietary advice, and fluid management. They should be informed how to monitor the condition at home and be advised when to call for help ('red flags'). These aspects promote patient autonomy, self-care, therapy adherence, and reduce the risk of inappropriate admission. Patient and carer support of at least moderate intensity is required at this stage as they come to terms with this new condition.

Phase 2

- Plateau period of variable duration representing an initial response to therapy.

Carer needs

Patient and carer education needs to be reinforced at intervals during this period as part of regular clinical review.

Phase 3

- Periods of instability linked to sudden functional deterioration or significant arrhythmia often requiring hospital admission.

Carer needs

Support needs to be increased and maintained at higher intensity in the face of overt disease progression.

Phase 4

Increasing symptoms and declining physical capacity, refractory to escalating HF treatment.

Carer needs

Full reassessment of carer needs as physical care requirements increase. Check understanding regarding aims of care and stage of illness.

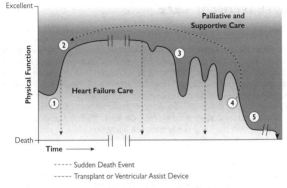

Fig. 15.1 HF disease trajectory. Reprinted from the *Journal of the American College of Cardiology*, Volume 54, Issue 5, Sarah J. Goodlin, Palliative Care in Congestive Heart Failure, 386–396, 2009, with permission from Elsevier.

Bereavement care

Despite the turbulence of the disease trajectory, many patients and carers may still not appreciate the likelihood of functional decline or the terminal nature of HF and when death occurs this is often felt to be unexpected and to come as a shock. Bereavement care should be incorporated within advanced HF care to support families and carers and reduce the risk of complicated grief reactions.[10] The Department of Health has produced guidelines to help structure bereavement services:[11]

- Achieving a 'good death' can aid carer adjustment in bereavement. Retrospective studies of carers have demonstrated that both dying at home and the dying experience not being perceived as protracted or distressing reduces the risks of carers developing bereavement problems.[12]

- Dealing with sudden death in the community demands particularly sensitive practical handling by the GP, the police, and the coroner's service. Carers exposed to the unfamiliar scenario of a sudden death may feel bewildered or guilty with a sense they have failed their loved one in the absence of the expertise or support routinely available in hospital.[13]

- The perception of the quality of death in hospital may be influenced by apparent discordance between the perceptions of patients', families', and health professionals' views of the goals of care. Conflicts may arise in families seeking 'only' comfort care while the patient is subjected to intrusive investigation or interventions when the situation appears to be futile. Conversely, conflicts may arise if patient and family are seeking ongoing interventions while health care professionals provide 'supportive care only'. Guidelines on care after sudden death in hospital have been published to help staff deal with these issues.[14]

- HF care is usually highly technical, and families may feel disempowered by the caring environment and a lack of comprehensible information. For their part, hospital staff, who are usually dealing with highly technical information, may feel less comfortable in dealing with other aspects of care. For example staff may be reluctant to broach issues of spiritual care, but access to faith leaders and participation in rituals by families with a religious belief can be very important at this time (see 📖 Chapter 14).

Perhaps the key skill in bereavement care is the very difficult task of diagnosing dying clearly and making sure that patient, family and carers are prepared and informed:

- Complicated grief is not always easy to anticipate and professional involvement too early on can disempower the family and social supports which are often of most value following on from a death. However, if adaptation to life following a bereavement is clearly not taking place, then referral to professional or voluntary services may be appropriate. Voluntary organizations such as Cruse Bereavement Care are also available to provide support (http://www.crusebereavementcare.org.uk/).

- After death, it is important to maintain contact with the family and thus reduce the sense of abandonment that is commonly felt. The hospital-based HF professional primarily involved with the patient, and the GP, should make contact with the family or caregivers, express condolences, and afford them the opportunity to ask questions and voice any concerns.

Supporting health professionals

It is also important to provide support to staff who may be affected by the death of a patient they have cared for over a prolonged period. Losing a patient after a long professional relationship may induce a sense of failure and feelings of professional inadequacy. Acknowledging such emotions is important as a coping mechanism and where possible the team should be afforded an opportunity for formal reflection.[15] Staff working in intensive care areas or palliative care may be particularly prone to emotional over-load leading to burnout or compassion fatigue and mechanisms should be in place to counsel such staff if appropriate.[16]

Support providers

Organizational support

- The BHF provides patient and carer support through more than 300 cardiac support groups across the country. There is also access to end of life care and bereavement support (http://www.bhf.org.uk/living-with-a-heart-condition/how-we-can-help-you/dealing-with-end-of-life.aspx).
- Patients can share their experiences through Hearty Voices (http://www.bhf.org.uk/heart-health/how-we-help/training/hearty-voices.aspx).
- The Heart Failure Association of the European Society of Cardiology has also developed a web-based information guide for those affected by HF. This includes a specific section dedicated to caregivers (http://www.heartfailurematters.org/EN/ForCaregivers/Pages/index.aspx).
- NHS Choices, Carers Direct: a web-based resource providing carers with information a variety of support (http://www.nhs.uk/CarersDirect/guide/kinds/Pages/Overview.aspx?WT.srch=1).
- The Carers UK website (http://www.carersuk.org/) gives excellent generic advice.

References

1 National Audit Office (2008) *End of life care*. National Audit Office, London (http://www.nao.org.uk/publications/0708/end_of_life_care.aspx).

2 Lang CC, Mancini DM (2007) Non-cardiac comorbidities in chronic heart failure. *Heart* **93**, 665–71.

3 Nordgren L, Sörensen S (2003) Symptoms experienced in the last six months of life in patients with end-stage heart failure. *Eur J Cardiovasc Nurs* **2**, 213–17.

4 Pattenden JF, Roberts H, Lewin RJP (2007) Living with heart failure: patient and carer perspectives. *Eur J Cardiovasc Nurs* **6**, 273–9.

5 Saunders MM (2008) Factors associated with caregiver burden in heart failure family caregivers. *Western J Nurs Res* **30**, 943–59.

6 Luttik ML, Jaarsma T, Veeger N, Tijssen J, Sanderman R, van Veldhuisen DJ (2007) Caregiver burden in partners of heart failure patients; limited influence of disease severity. *Eur J Heart Fail* **9**, 695–701.

7 Tomassini C, Glaser K, Wolf DA, Broese van Groenou MI, Grundy E (2004) Living arrangements among older people: an overview of trends in Europe and the USA. *Popul Trends* **115**, 24–34.

8 Department of Health (2010) *Building a national care service*. (http://www.dh.gov.uk/prod_consum_dh/groups/dh_digitalassets/documents/digitalasset/dh_114923.pdf).

9 Gott M, Barnes S, Parker C et al. (2007) Dying trajectories in heart failure. *Palliat Med* **21**, 95–9.

10 National Cancer Institute. *Complicated grief*. (http://www.nci.nih.gov/cancertopics/pdq/supportivecare/bereavement/Patient/page8) accessed 10 July 2010.

11 Department of Health (2005) *When a patient dies: advice on developing bereavement services in the NHS* (http://www.dh.gov.uk/en/Publicationsandstatistics/Publications/PublicationsPolicyAndGuidance/DH_4122191).

12 Small N, Barnes S, Gott M et al. (2009) Dying, death and bereavement: a qualitative study of the views of carers of people with heart failure in the UK. *BMC Palliat Care* **8**:6 doi: 10.1186/1472-684X-8-6.

13 Department of Health (2008) *End of life care strategy*, Department of Health, London. Available at: http://www.cpa.org.uk/cpa/End_of_Life_Care_Strategy.pdf

14 Frost PJ, Leadbeatter S, Wise MP (2010) Managing sudden death in hospital. *BMJ* **340**, 1024–8.

15 Goodlin SJ, Cassell EJ (2008) Coping with patients' deaths. In: *Supportive care in heart failure* (ed. J Beattie, S Goodlin), pp. 477–82. Oxford University Press, Oxford.

16 Sandgren A, Thulesius H, Fridlund B, Petersson K (2006) Striving for emotional survival in palliative cancer nursing. *Qual Health Res* **16**, 79–96.

Index